THE EGO DIET

THE EGO DIET

Gerald Laurence

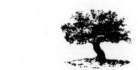

Oak Tree Publications, Inc.
San Diego, California

To Midge, who should know that part of my love
for her daughter is hers as well

Published by Oak Tree

Distributed in the United States by
Oak Tree Publications, Inc.
San Diego, California

Library of Congress Cataloging in Publication Data

Laurence, Gerald, 1948–
     The ego diet.

     1. Reducing diets.   2. Reducing--Psychological
aspects.   I. Title.
RM222.2.L36   1984   613.2'5   84-16635

ISBN 0-916392-005-5

First Edition
1 2 3 4 5 6 7 8 9 88 87 86 85 84
Printed and bound in the United States of America

Contents

A Word Of Caution

EVERY diet is dangerous for somebody. Indeed, every food is potentially harmful to someone. You may have allergies to some foods. You may have blood-sugar abnormalities or suffer from diabetes or hypoglycemia.

Because of this, the author cannot assume any liability resulting from the application of the principles outlined in this book. The plans in *The Ego Diet* have been thoroughly researched and have been used by many people over several years. They have been found to work without causing any ill effects. Still, you must find out about your body's needs from a physician before attempting a change in your diet.

Please consult your doctor.

Starring You!

YOU are the hero of this book. Every word is written just for you, and every piece of advice is presented with you in mind.

Naturally, the best interests of you and your body are at the center of everything in The Ego Diet. Still, in order to have a hero—you—there must also be a villain. And the villain might also be you, because what you do with the advice in this book will determine whether or not you reach a happy ending: in other words, whether or not you are able to reach and maintain your best weight and appearance.

But don't worry. You know you can do it; you *can* be the hero.

Are you the right person for The Ego Diet?

Are you a man or woman who is concerned about looking and feeling your best? Are you interested in finding a diet plan that extends your current diet and makes it easier to live with? Do you want to maintain your weight with ease?

If you answered yes to any of these questions, The Ego Diet is perfect for you. It is the one diet plan that complements and accompanies other diet plans. And it is the one diet plan that is easily extended throughout the foreseeable future.

Not just for people who are overweight

Do you want to maintain your present weight? Do you want to find a way to motivate yourself to stay on your current diet? Do you want to "psych yourself up" to continue healthy eating habits and exercise?

Great. The Ego Diet is ideal for men and women who are already at their perfect weight and size.

What about the overweight and obese?

Lots of people are overweight. Many are actually obese (there is a technical definition that relates to the percentage of body fat, but we'll just leave it at that).

Some overweight people have no interest in dieting. Let's just ignore them. Some others have given up trying to do anything about it. This is a mistake. The human body was not meant to carry around extra folds of flab, and if you do it for too long, you could reduce your life expectancy because of any number of weight-related ailments. Heart disease is one of them.

No matter what you think, being overweight is very rarely the result of a glandular or metabolic problem. It is not simply a problem of getting older. Nor is it the result of your genes. True, there are people with biological or other problems that cause obesity, and your doctor can tell you if you are one of those. But in the main, it's usually one's own fault if the scale tips too high.

Men: Do you feel afraid to diet?

Many men do not admit to going on a diet. Many others are actually fearful of trying to change eating patterns. The reason for this probably has to do with the association of diets with physicians' recommendations regarding the avoidance of cardiac problems, diabetes, and other health problems. In books and films these recommendations are very often shown as being made to older men. Therefore, young and middle-aged men, afraid others will think they are getting old, are reluctant to admit they are on a diet.

This is nonsense. It's partly the reason The Ego Diet was invented. The Ego Diet stresses a positive approach to dieting so that it becomes known as the healthy diet, or even the young person's diet (young at heart, that is—The Ego Diet may be used by youngsters of 65 and older, too).

Another problem with men and diets comes from those *macho* types who tend to guzzle beer and stuff their faces with junk food after eating salads with sprouts at their exercise spa. These guys give dieting a bad name with their "drink by night and jog by day" routine. And besides, they're only doing it to attract potential bed-partners. Hmmm, but then, that's one of the results of successfully following The Ego Diet, so perhaps they're on the right track after all.

Women: How many diets have you tried?

If you're like most women, you've been on many diets. Some worked, some didn't work, and some would have worked if you could have put up with them for a while. You've also probably purchased other diet books. But no matter what diets you've tried, you've gained back whatever pounds you've lost.

Right now, you'd like to lose a few of those pounds. You want a flatter stomach. You want slimmer hips. You want arms and inner thighs that don't shake with extra flesh. You're not fat, but you know you could look a lot better just by losing a little weight. Or, perhaps you only need to tone up your muscles a bit—to redistribute your weight slightly. And then maybe you're one of the lucky ones who have managed to attain your perfect weight, but you very much want to maintain it.

Whichever it is you wish to achieve, The Ego Diet is going to help you, scientifically.

How men and women benefit from the ego and The Ego Diet

If other diets fail, and exercise programs only take off a small percentage of weight, and if you gain back what you lose, then what makes The Ego Diet work for you?

Every man and woman has a psychological attribute in the mind and soul called the ego. It is the thinking and feeling self that keeps you from sinking to the level of animals. It is what keeps you aware of yourself in relation to others. The ego also keeps you aware of your own needs, desires, and wants.

In the psychological theories of Freud, there are three entities: the id, the superego, and the ego. The *id* is part of your unconscious, which holds your basic impulses and desires. The *superego* may be roughly called your conscience, which is opposed to the id. And the *ego* seeks to maintain a balance between the two.

The ego thus becomes your central driving force in most actions. You might think of the ego as a control tower from which your body checks on the outside world to see what must be done to steer a proper course through the day. No matter how pressing are the needs of the id, and no matter how repressive are the responses of the superego, it is the ego that is in control. And you can use this mysterious and powerful control to help you lose weight.

I say mysterious because no one knows for certain just how the ego operates. Entire books have been written about it. Philosophically, the ego has been argued about and discussed for years. In psychology, entire schools of thought have debated—sometimes quite violently—about the ego. The point is, the ego is one of the most powerful intangible objects on earth.

The Ego Diet is designed to harness the immense power of the ego in a manner that helps you. Your ego can work for you if you let it. You just need some guidelines as to how to think about food and drink, and as to what to do when buying food or drink.

It almost doesn't matter what these guidelines are called. I have called them The Ego Diet, but there are many sophisticated methods of procedure.

For example, Joseph Wolpe developed a behavior modification technique called systematic desensitization therapy. In this method, people are urged to associate pleasing feelings with situations they normally have trouble handling. Another example is Abraham H. Maslow's theory of motivation, which is based on a hierarchy of needs—the idea that basic needs (like shelter, sustenance, and water) must be satisfied before you move on to the next higher level of needs. This can be applied to dieting by treating basic foods separately from "fun" foods like sweets, and by finding a balance between the two.

These and many other psychological methods will work to help you, but The Ego Diet incorporates a great many of the underlying principles in these methods. The Ego Diet is also, frankly, easier to read, simpler to follow, and a lot more fun.

While the psychological and physiological principles incorporated into The Ego Diet are not themselves covered in this book, the bibliography will lead you to material discussing each subject in detail.

You will succeed on The Ego Diet

With The Ego Diet, you will lose weight, maintain your ideal weight, feel better, and look more attractive. And you will be able to continue to do so easier than ever before because you will be compelled to succeed by the force of your own ego.

You've got what it takes

You know it because you can feel it. It's been there inside you for many years.

How many times have you said to yourself, "I'm different, I'm special, I'm better . . ." or even "I'm worth it . . ."?

You've probably said these things to yourself hundreds or even thousands of times.

Perhaps you said things like this more when you were younger—when you were growing up. Or you may find you are saying them more now. Either way, you are having to fight against the pressures of the world. You're subjected to quite a lot of brainwashing in your encounters with other people. The most upsetting encounters are with so-called mature people—the kind who make others feel inferior. It's enough to make you want to drop out of society.

However, even if you were to remove yourself from contact with other human beings, you'd probably still be bombarded with the images and sounds of these people via radio, TV, newspapers, and magazines. (And if you were to remove yourself from these things, what would be left for you to do?)

The problem is this: we are all told

- ► how to look,
- ► how to feel,
- ► how to act.

It may be implied, but it is still there, in commercials, in popular fiction, in the movies, on the TV talk shows. You can look at The Ego Diet as a way to fight back against this brainwashing—and as a way to look and feel great at the same time. That should make you feel special.

You're right to feel special

You *are* special. People are looking at you. They look up to you because of who you are and what you are (or because of the potential you display).

You're either famous (or about to be famous) or you're well known in your field (or about to become well known). Or you're simply very interested in getting certain other people to become involved with you. Or even all of the above.

In every instance in that list, people look to you and at you. So you want to make certain you look and feel your best at every hour of the day.

Because of this, The Ego Diet is tailor-made for you. If you have to set an example for others, The Ego Diet is perfect for you. If others depend on you, it's perfect for you. In short, if you want to get total control of your life, then The Ego Diet is one means to that end.

You needn't be afraid of stressing your ego

Your ego is not to be feared. Or ignored (although you couldn't do that even if you tried). Unfortunately, it has become unfashionable to stress your own needs. We are supposed to talk and act as if we are not self-oriented and self-actualized.

In this regard, the ego has taken a bum rap. The only possible problem associated with the ego is when it isn't being used—when the selfish, lustful id takes over or when the prissy, uptight superego takes over. Your ego is a normal, healthy part of you and you should use it. The Ego Diet is simply a way to channel some of the power of your ego into a specific useful area.

The Ego Diet works with you

With most chapters in this book, you will find a new, simple method for dieting and maintaining your best looks. Every method actually uses the compelling nature of your own ego as a starting point.

By relying on the internal mechanism of your own ego, you will obtain more reinforcement to remain on your diet than with any other diet plan.

Many diets ask you to do lots of things you would not do naturally. The Ego Diet primarily relies on changing your *learned* behavior while leaving untouched your inner, natural drives and desires.

There are already many people benefiting from this aspect of this diet. They are in various cities across the United States, and there will soon be many many more of them across the world. All the people I know who have followed any one of the methods outlined in this book have benefited from it. And their own egos were the guiding force in their transformations.

It's for every body type

According to the body-type theory, people are divided into three basic types:

- ► Ectomorph (ecto = without; morph = shape), *a thin person*
- ► Mesomorph (meso = intermediate), *an athletic person*
- ► Endomorph (endo = within), *a fat person*

This theory, called constitutional psychology, was developed by William Sheldon in the 1930s. Although there has been some controversy concerning how Sheldon assigned particular personality traits to individuals with the different body types, it is still true that each of us tends to be like one of the three basic types.

There are certain problems associated with each body type. The ectomorph, or thin person, does not eat enough or burns off food through worry or other activity. Further, smaller amounts of food and alcohol will affect thinner people more quickly.

The mesomorph, or athletic person, must maintain muscle tone, must get enough fuel food, and must not eat too much prior to physical exertion.

The endomorph, or fat person, simply eats too much, too often, and usually eats the wrong foods. All this, coupled with a lack of proper exercise, makes such a person a candidate for heart disease.

All three body types can be aided by The Ego Diet. You can even change from one body type to another.

Proof

I have benefited from The Ego Diet. When I posed for a magazine advertisement for a manufacturer of computer support equipment, my flabby face bore a strong resemblance to an overinflated soccer ball.

Now, despite my having entered what is somewhat unfetchingly called middle age, most agree that I appear to the world as a more firm, taut, and streamlined individual. I feel stronger, healthier, and happier, too. And what's more important, The Ego Diet keeps on helping me stay this way.

A different diet every day?

The Ego Diet offers enormous variety and flexibility. Its various diet plans can be used in a great many ways.

What's more, these different plans are for the most part interchangeable. As you'll see, you can use The Ego Diet one way on Monday, another on Tuesday, and so on throughout the week.

And, of course, you may find one part of it to stick with for a long time.

What The Ego Diet can't do

You will look better, feel better, and live longer by staying with the proper diet, but there is no way any mere diet can prevent hair loss, extend your youth, cure any psychosomatic disorders, or clear up any sexual dysfunction.

To the extent that The Ego Diet helps you enjoy life, you'll feel as if you're staying young, and that should help you live longer and avoid problems in bed.

A word of caution

A physician's care and guidance is advisable when attempting physiological alterations such as may occur with a change in your diet.

Prudence and common sense should enable you to mix and match the various Ego Diet procedures without any problem. However, when in doubt, see your doctor. After all, it may be that you have suffered from weight problems for years due to allergic reactions to foods, or for any of a dozen other reasons. The Ego Diet can work very well with your physician's instructions, but only a fool would attempt to go against a doctor's orders. So, please consult your physician about your diet plans.

Feel better and look better!

Those are your goals. The various Ego Diet methods outlined in this book are your road maps. Not every one of the methods will work for you 100 percent of the time. Most of them will have some beneficial effect, and some of them will turn out to be your main avenues to lifelong weight management.

But the best thing about The Ego Diet is your being able and free to switch from one method to another as the need or whim suits you.

For example, if the ways of using water to help your diet (Chapter 10) don't work for you at this particular time, don't worry about it. Just move back to the mirror method (Chapter 3).

By the same token, if the mirror method doesn't work every time you need it, then the pinch procedure (Chapter 5) might be just the thing for you.

You're completely free to skip around in The Ego Diet. This freedom makes your whole approach to weight loss and weight maintenance much more interesting. It also enables you to concentrate on only certain portions of the book.

You can easily leave some methods alone altogether, or simply save them for future use. In a pinch, perhaps.

If you read only one chapter, but find in it something that makes so much sense for you—something that truly takes hold of your own ego drive—great! That's all you may need of this book! You can then save the remainder of The Ego Diet for several years down the road, just in case.

What matters is for you to get to the weight you want, stay at that weight, and feel great about yourself the entire time.

Whatever method works best for you and keeps you healthy is fine. That is why I have provided as many facets to The Ego Diet as could reasonably be included in this volume.

2

You're On A Diet Even If You Deny It

STRICTLY speaking, everybody is on a diet. And you're on that diet all the time. Your diet consists of whatever you eat on a regular basis.

This concept scares some people, but most find it a great relief. At last, you don't have to be worried about "going on a diet"—you're already on one. All you have to do is modify your current diet.

Just as the word "ego" has gotten a bum rap lately, so has the word "diet." There has been so much attention paid to diets, diet plans, and just plain diet fads that the term sometimes causes a knee-jerk reaction: "Oh no, not another diet!"

The big problem with the word "diet" is that it is most often used to describe the *control* of your eating habits. While it is true that The Ego Diet also seeks to provide control of your eating, with The Ego Diet *you* are in control. This is unlike many other diet programs which preach and proscribe.

With The Ego Diet, *self*-control of your eating patterns is of primary importance. Still, as in every diet plan, the things you will control are: how much food you eat, how often you eat, when you eat, and what kinds of foods are eaten.

Eating beyond your needs (or eating and ignoring your needs)

An aging football player who has stopped training but who has kept the same eating habits as when he was very active in the sport may eat enough food every day for six of your regular meals. A diet like that, even if comprised of the right foods eaten at sensible times during the day, consists of much more food than necessary. And, since the intake of food is too high, added pounds will be the result.

To take the reverse situation, consider a young woman suffering from anorexia. Over a two-day period, she may eat as little as one of your meals. Again, no matter that what she eats is from the four basic food groups, a diet like that will produce starvation. Hospitalization—if she's lucky—will be the result.

In both of these examples, however, a diet was being followed. Not a healthy diet. Not a wise diet. But a diet nonetheless. The word diet does not have to refer to a regimented and restricted intake of food. If you eat sweet rolls in the morning, hamburgers at noon, and meat and potatoes at night, your diet consists of starch and fatty meats. Without fruits and vegetables, you'll soon be susceptible to illness. It's hard to believe sane people would continue with such eating habits, yet they do. And each is still on a diet, no matter how unwise and unhealthy it is.

The problem most of us face is finding the right diet for our needs. You don't always need a large amount of food to satisfy your body's demands for fuel. Nor do you always need to limit yourself to very small amounts of food in order to lose weight. The idea is to meet your body's needs without eating more than necessary. When you eat beyond your needs, you add inches to your waist, your arms, your thighs, your rump, and so on. Or, if you simply eat the wrong foods *all the time*, you can wind up depriving your body of vitamins and protein.

By thinking of yourself and your body's needs, you will be more likely to make the right decisions regarding what you eat, when you eat, and how often you eat. The beauty of The Ego Diet is that it stresses the act of thinking of yourself and your own needs, and that helps you eat right.

Think of yourself

That's the right thing to do: Think only of yourself when it comes to food. Don't worry about making those other people at the dinner table "comfortable" by ordering a big meal just like they do. Don't be pressured into having the full course dinner—order what you want.

Don't think about how pleasing it will be for your host when you accept a second helping. Just refuse as politely as possible. Either that, or make certain your "firsts" are small enough to allow you to have "seconds."

Don't load up your plate in the buffet line just to "be one of the boys" or to go along with the crowd. Take just what you want and ignore the urging of others around you.

Remember—you're on The Ego Diet. That means you're the person in charge; you're the one in control. Don't be bashful about it, just speak right up. Go ahead and announce to everybody that you are the person controlling your own eating habits and you'll thank them to butt out. Be polite, but be firm. (One of the nice side benefits to stating that you're using The Ego Diet is that it also announces to the world that *you* are the one controlling your life.)

"What can you eat on The Ego Diet?"

You'll get asked that question quite often. And you'll be able to answer, "Anything *I* decide to eat, because on The Ego Diet, I'm the one who controls which foods are eaten, when I eat them, and how much of each I eat." Perhaps you won't word it exactly like that, but you'll be able to point out that The Ego Diet, unlike most other diet plans, leaves you in command. With this freedom, however, comes some responsibility.

If you have answered "no" to an offer of a certain kind of food you decide shouldn't be eaten at that moment, that really means *no!* Not "maybe," or "perhaps," or "I'm saying 'no,' but go ahead and convince me to try it." It means *n-o*, no. Do not be forced into having something you've already refused.

You can be as polite as you wish about it, even saying something like "no thanks, not right now; maybe later." But if you decline something, make it clear to your friends that you really mean it. After all, since you are the most important person in the world, your decision about what foods you eat had damn well better be respected. If it isn't respected, excuse yourself and depart. Go graciously, but go. The worst friends someone on a diet can have are people who are compulsive eaters, especially those who like to convince everyone around them to join in the foodfest. (Often the only reason they want you to eat what they're eating is to lessen their own guilt about breaking their own diet plans. Just because they aren't strong enough, just because they lack the self-respect you're developing for yourself, is no reason for you to be sucked down to their level.)

Usually, however, people will be interested in talking about The Ego Diet with you. "What do you mean you can eat anything you decide to eat?" they'll ask. "Aren't there restricted lists of foods, meals, drink, and so on?"

Nope. The Ego Diet isn't like other diets. Common usage these days has it that a diet refers to specific, rigid requirements: lists of foods, lists of food groups, lists of exact portions or amounts of food that must be

followed in each meal . . . and these lists have to be adhered to for certain definite periods of time in order to accomplish certain changes
(inches on your waistline, pounds on a scale, and so on). People have
come to expect this kind of restriction because of the way they view
diets themselves. People usually go on a diet only to accomplish certain
things—and they doom themselves to almost certain failure because of
these things. Here are the reasons usually given for going on a diet:

"My doctor told me to."
> Already, this person isn't in full control because the diet is
> imposed from without rather than from within.

"I've got to lose some weight."
> Not a bad idea in itself, but the goal should be to attain your
> ideal weight and maintain it, not just to lose some weight.

"I'm having my picture taken and want to look thinner."
> Again, the wrong goal—a diet should be used to look and feel
> your best through your life, not just for a one-time event.

"I'm going on a date to the beach and I want to fit into my suit."
> Wrong again—one-time events are very likely to destroy any
> chance for staying at your best weight.

"I'm getting in shape for the 5K run."
> Well, this might be okay *if* you're already at your "cruising
> weight" and you simply want to put yourself on an extra protein
> diet, but it's foolhardy if you're out of shape to begin with.

I could go on and on with this list. You could add a whole bunch of
good lines you've overheard or even used yourself. All of these reasons
reaffirm one of the bigger problems with what are usually called diets:
People only consider diets a necessary evil to be endured for as short a
period of time as possible.

That is the wrong way to think about diets.

The problem of "diets"

By following rules, lists, formulae, tables, charts, diagrams, and
pictures to control your eating, you're limiting yourself to unrealistic—
and sometimes unhealthful—diet plans. More often than not, all of the
above is made even worse by putting some sort of arbitrary time limit
on the dieting plan.

Going along with that type of diet program practically guarantees the
diet will fail. Even if you lose weight under such a regimented system,

what happens when you go off the diet? Right—you gain back all the weight you just lost.

This problem is resolved by The Ego Diet. By using certain psychological behavior modification techniques and several other psychologically based methods, The Ego Diet will put you in charge of your eating, in charge of your body, and in charge of your life.

You can stay on The Ego Diet—with ease

Instead of limiting you to blindly following charts, lists, and tables— and instead of limiting you to certain brief time periods for dieting—The Ego Diet asks you to have a positive outlook about your dieting, to trust and rely on your own ability to judge what and when to eat. With the right outlook about yourself and your body (and a brief glance at this book from time to time), you will be able to keep on The Ego Diet for the rest of your life, and enjoy it!

What was that? Yes, you read that correctly. It does sound rather dreadful at first: "Stay on a diet the rest of my life? That would be terrible." But it's actually the other way around. It's much more horrible to go on a diet, then off it, then on another one, then off it . . . and so on. You know the old joke: "How many pounds have you lost so far?" asks one person. "Oh, about 3,956 pounds," is the reply. "How much have you gained back?" is the next question. "Roughly forty-one hundred. So far."

It's also somewhat dangerous to lose weight, gain it back, lose it-gain it-lose it, over and over again. Cholesterol, a fatty alcohol which comes principally from bile, increases in your blood when you gain weight. Fatty deposits from the cholesterol become wedged in your arteries. When you lose weight, these fatty deposits do not reduce in the same proportion as your weight loss. Therefore, each time you gain weight and lose it again, your blood vessels get narrower. Every bit of narrowing increases your chances for a heart attack.

Stress

Other diets are much more difficult than The Ego Diet because you have to keep going back to them over and over again. In addition to the cholesterol problem mentioned above, a tremendous amount of psychological stress may be experienced in the start-up phase of any diet, even one you've been on before. By keeping on a diet-management plan like that offered by The Ego Diet, you only have to go through the start-up period once.

No matter how well-intentioned you are at the start of any new diet, you know from bitter experience how easy it is to "fall off" your plan after just a few days. (I once fell off a new diet after only two hours.)

Here's where The Ego Diet saves you time and trouble. With it, you will be able to vary your eating habits to a great extent. Plus, you will be able to alter the way you approach all your meals (and often the way you set up a meal makes all the difference in determining the amount and kind of food you eat).

Once you make the commitment to follow the basic outline of The Ego Diet, you have only to perform some very simple "reminders" to yourself in order to stay on the diet. And since these reminders all stem from your basic need to feel good about yourself (your ego at work, here), you are much more likely to perform the reminders over and over again without even thinking about it. "Falling off" the diet is something that doesn't happen, because there is no horrible, big, diet bandwagon to fall off—there are no lists of foods to eat, no lists of foods to avoid, no calories to count, no scales to stand on—there are only those ego reminders you make for yourself.

You have enough "will power"

You don't have to worry about your will power. It doesn't matter what may have happened in the past; those diets you tried before didn't have the right psychological approach to your will power. Whatever it is that you need in the area of will, you've got it! You've proven that you're a special person capable of great things—you've proven it to yourself, and now you're going to prove it to the world. That's why you've selected something that sounds as outrageous as The Ego Diet.

Part of the success of The Ego Diet even comes from the name. It sounds great. Think about telling your friends: "Me? Oh, I'm using The Ego Diet. It's the only one that gives me enough different approaches to control my own impulses and to take full control of my body and its needs." You can just imagine the look on your friends' faces when you tell them that (although you should be certain, for maximum effect, that you've already lost some weight before making your announcement).

Avoid "that look"

Since we're on the subject of the look on the faces of your friends, let me reveal something I have never before told to anyone.

Several years ago, before discovering The Ego Diet, I had been coasting through life, eating just for the taste of food rather than the fuel content. I had shunned every form of exercise, preferring to stay in bed as much as possible. I used elevators even if I only had to go up or down one flight of stairs. I took the car instead of walking even if I only needed to go down to the corner drugstore. And, of course, I was very fond of eating all manner of foods at all hours of the day or night.

I was even more rounded than in that picture of me posing for that computer equipment ad.

A friend who knew me in college telephoned me at work, thinking of me as the svelte young man she went out with a few times. Now, my voice hadn't gotten fat or slothful, and our conversation proceeded nicely, leading me to conclude that an evening's reunion might have quite pleasurable consequences for both of us.

The date was made and I rushed home to change out of my suit, which was redolently reminiscent of the cigarettes people smoke in office buildings. And I took a shower. And I carefully selected my clothes. And I left early so as to be able to find where she was staying in plenty of time (I even took along a magazine, which I leafed through to kill time when it turned out that her place was easy to locate). And all the while, the most delicious anticipation was driving me crazy inside.

I kept remembering the shape of her legs, the curve of her neck, the quickness of her smile, the sparkle of her laugh, the daintiness of her waist. I also remembered her perfume, a lovely, longing, haunting scent that would stay with me for hours after leaving her side.

In short, I was making myself regret all the time we'd wasted since parting at college.

The hour of our reacquaintance arrived at last. I heaved myself out of the car, waddled up the steps, rang the bell, put a jaunty grin on my wide face as she opened the door, and . . . I watched in horror as her face betrayed her disappointment at the fact that there was so much more of me standing in front of her. Apparently, there was too much of me for her to contemplate for long.

Needless to say, the evening turned out to be considerably less exciting than my hyperactive imagination had set me up to expect. The shock and shame of that terrifying moment stayed with me all the way home. Indeed, it remained with me for quite some time afterward. Now, I use that moment as a last-ditch reminder if I really need a jolt to stay on The Ego Diet.

That's just the sort of thing The Ego Diet relies upon: the workings of your own mind, your own emotions, and your own feelings.

The Ego Diet doesn't involve tape measures. It doesn't involve pills. It involves *you*. That's why it's different, and that's why it will work.

Ask yourself . . .

Do you think about yourself and your well-being? Of course you do. That's why The Ego Diet is so powerful: it uses your own self-interest.

Do you have the ability to go back on another kind of diet? Of course you do. You know you can do it, and you know you can lose weight. You've lost weight in the past, and you can do it again.

The difference now is that The Ego Diet will give you the drive and the power to remain on your diet and keep off those unneeded pounds you currently desire to lose.

The Ego Diet will give you the strength and courage to maintain your optimum weight and your ideal figure.

Please believe in yourself and read on. Your first step has already been taken.

Now comes the fun part.

3

The Mirror Method

MIRRORS are magical. In addition to all the normal, everyday things for which you rely on them—to see how your clothes look on you, to comb your hair, brush your teeth, shave, put on make-up, and so on—mirrors are also something very special.

They are an excellent tool to help you lose weight and then maintain your proper weight.

Try this experiment

Stand in front of a full-length mirror at home, alone. Take off all your clothes. Right, all of them. Now, look at your reflection.

Okay, let's take stock.

This is what your lover sees. Is it what you want him or her to see?

Look at your waist. Your hips. Your belly. Your arms. Your legs. Your chest.

Turn around and look at yourself over your shoulder. Look at the area between your shoulders and below your neck. This is an area of the body many people overlook. Is it hunched and flabby? If so, it could be because your back isn't being held straight. Turn sideways to check your posture. You might find that you can look five pounds lighter and thinner just by stopping your slouching. Good—do it. When you walk around during the day, imagine yourself an inch or so taller than you are, and hold yourself erect to maintain that tallness.

This is not cheating. It's not cheating on your diet. And it's not cheating on your friends. If you look as if you've lost five pounds, then you've as good as lost them.

The Ego Diet mirror method helps you in this very simple way: you look into mirrors to find out how your image relates to what you want it to be. Mirrors can be your *reminders* to eat better, exercise more, and so on. All you're doing at the moment, however, is finding out what simple things you can do to alter your appearance for the better.

"Thinking yourself taller" and adopting better, healthier posture are legitimate ways to look thinner and better. Both can be easily and quickly monitored throughout the day with mirrors. So go ahead and do either one or both.

Posture and mental attitude

I realize this is going to sound like a Pollyanna platitude, but you can also appear more vibrant just by "psyching yourself up." It's easy. Just throw back your head—shoulders, too—while keeping your backbone straight. Be sure to check in the mirror whether or not you need to tuck your bottom in and under while you stand or walk (it's a problem for many people, including me). One other thing: put a smile on your face. Now, stride—don't slouch—to your next meeting.

It works. Really! It's one reason why dancers work out in front of mirrors. Closely watching one's weight, form, and posture is an everyday part of a dancer's world. It should be part of yours, too. The amazing thing about checking yourself in the mirror to see if you're smiling and standing upright is that you actually do begin to feel better and happier. You'll also feel more confident. Remember the scenes in the film *All That Jazz* where Roy Scheider, playing director Bob Fosse's alter ego, psychs himself up each morning? He finishes getting dressed, looks himself straight in the eye in the bathroom mirror, and intones the, for him, magic words, "It's showtime, folks." Something like that can work for you, and you don't have to do it only in the morning.

When you walk out on the street, check out your posture in store window reflections or car window reflections. It'll help you.

Don't worry about the stories you've heard concerning people becoming "egomaniacs" because they turned too much toward themselves. You're not altering your attitudes about other people, only about yourself in relation to your own body. Forget about that mythological tale about Narcissus, the man who fell in love with his own reflection. It makes a nice story, but it didn't actually occur; it's a myth, remember. Besides, you've got plenty of other people-images in your life with whom you can fall in love (or you soon will have plenty of them!).

The stretch

When you feel yourself getting worn down during the day, find a mirror to pause in front of, and take a half a minute to stretch. Even if you can't get in front of a mirror, you can still do the stretch itself.

The full stretch is best: bend over at the waist, letting your arms dangle. Then, slowly raise yourself up, lifting your arms toward the ceiling as you rise. Try to feel your back straightening and lengthening as you lift your arms. Go on tiptoe; try to stretch out to actually touch the ceiling (one friend of mine likes to do this in a room with a very low ceiling so that he can touch the roof). Arch your back and then straighten it out and tuck your rump in and under. Now bring your arms down and come back off tiptoe. This exercise is similar to that performed by cats after taking a nap.

If you're with other people and can't do the full stretch, just throw back your arms, elbows first, and your shoulders. Rotate your head and neck. You can even do this sitting down, but be certain to keep your backbone straight. Give the other people in the room a big grin while you do it (you may feel a bit self-conscious the first few times you do the stretch, so the grin will come easy).

By doing the stretch at least once a day, you'll find that you go through your day with less fatigue. Your mental outlook will improve, too.

To make it a habit, however, give yourself a stretch and a grin (even if tiny ones) whenever you catch sight of yourself in a mirror. Or, you might want to do it just when you pass one particular mirror. Keep on doing this and you'll not only feel better and be more mentally alert, but you'll appear to have lost weight as well.

Don't fear your image

I know we started out with a frightening exercise (stripping in front of a mirror), but that's just part of the shock-therapy portion of The Ego Diet mirror method; the grinning and stretching are part of the cure, too, and you'll have to admit that they're a lot more fun.

It is still a good idea to keep stripping in front of a mirror as often as you need it (once a week is needed for some people, but even once a month is quite beneficial). Do it when you feel light and leaner than usual. That way, your image is a bit of encouragement to keep going. Remember, your image in the mirror is what you display to those with whom you're intimate. If you don't like what you see, then they might not like it either. If you're in doubt about their opinion, ask them. You might be surprised to learn that you've lost just enough weight to become more attractive to them even though you may still feel you have a way to go. In this happy event, you need only maintain your current weight. Do not try to lose a little more so that you have "a little room to gain back some weight if you feel like it." Do not try to go up and down in weight once you have reached your ideal weight.

When you ask your partner about your weight, you must not be offended if he or she thinks you could stand to lose or redistribute a few pounds. Getting upset about your weight is not going to help you and getting upset with loved ones isn't going to help any part of your life. Besides, if you ask a question about yourself while using The Ego Diet —a diet that stresses your own inner power—you've got to accept the answer no matter how unflattering it may be. After all, you're accepting the view you display for yourself in the mirror, aren't you? So, you've got to accept the truth about the way you look through someone else's eyes. If you want to avoid problems with other people's opinions, just keep your thoughts and questions to yourself.

Helpful hints

You can use the mirror to help yourself appear thinner in other ways. Take your clothing, for example. It's odd that many people "look but don't see" when they examine their clothing in a mirror. The advice I'm about to give may seem old hat to you, but judging from the way many people dress, there's nothing old hat about the following hints:

▶ Solids usually make you look slimmer than prints; dark colors are usually more slimming than light colors.

▶ Stripes, while not as slimming as most solids, are better than most prints; horizontal stripes make you look wider; vertical stripes do tend to make you look taller, but beware of the "barber pole" effect when the stripes are too thick.

▶ We all have certain outfits that make us feel good and these outfits almost always are the ones that are the most flattering; if you could get your whole wardrobe to have that effect, you'd always look better and thinner; on days when you're feeling a bit down, slip into those "up" clothes—it'll help.

▶ We all have skin tone and hair color that look better in combination with certain colors of clothing; basically, you look your best in colors that are associated with one of the four seasons, spring, fall, winter, or summer.

"Seasonal" colors

Like most of us, you've probably purchased clothes in many different colors. And you've probably done so with little or no regard for how the color might bring out your skin tone, preferring to rely on such things as "this will go with those shoes," or "red always looks good with my hair," and so on. But are you really sure about what colors go well with your pigmentation?

Go to your closet and select some clothes from each of the four seasonal color groups:

▶ Spring colors: pastels in peach, lime green, etc.; baby pink, baby blue, etc. Remember spring colors as "a breath of color," or a hint of color—the way flowers look prior to blooming.

▶ Summer colors: a fuller range of flower colors, from pink to rose red, from iris blue to dark blue, from pale yellow to deep yellow, etc. Summer colors include the flower colors in all their glory.

▶ Fall colors: golds, browns, orange, olive, khaki, beige, etc. Fall colors are like the leaves turning on the trees just before falling.

▶ Winter colors: white, ice blue, steel blue, gray, etc. Winter colors are like a snow-and-ice-covered countryside.

Now hold up clothes from each category in turn while studying yourself in the mirror. Notice how some tend to make you look heavier, larger, more washed-out, and less alive? And see how others tend to make you appear more vibrant as well as slimmer and more attractive?

Take note of which are *your* colors and begin weeding out those things in your wardrobe that do not help your appearance.

Hair

It's probably worth it to find somebody who is excellent at shaping or "sculpting" hair and pay whatever it may cost for a first-rate styling. By all means take in photos of people with hairstyles you admire, but be realistic about it. Study your image and compare it with the photos you intend to take. Do the people in the photos have the same shape head? The same coloring of hair and skin? The same type of hair? (It's difficult to determine whether someone in a photo has oily or dry hair, but you can sometimes tell if they have fine or thick hair, and you can usually tell if they have a lot of it left!) Ask your stylist for advice. Stylists want you to look great so that people compliment you. That makes you want to come back.

When in doubt, go for the more conservative hairstyle. You look thinner when you don't call attention to yourself with trendy, faddish styles.

Put up more mirrors

Women don't seem to have a problem about mirrors, but men sometimes need to have more of them around. (I'm not suggesting men are less vain than women—far from it—it's just that society puts pressure on men not to pay as much attention to mirrors in public, although this restriction is lifted in the case of teenagers and their rearview mirrors.)

Remember to *study* yourself in the mirror. Make a special effort to do so prior to eating anything. Pause for reflection (sorry about that one) before each meal. Think back to what you saw when you removed your clothes. Tell yourself that you can only change your image through your own will power at the table. Keep your stripping image in mind as you order your meals and as you eat them. If this helps you order a more sensible meal, then the mirror method is working for you.

You might find that the mental picture of yourself during the stripping session isn't as effective as the feeling you get when you're thinking yourself taller. You can easily use the more positive taller-is-thinner approach. Often, people tell me the good feelings they get from the stretch can be a help when at the dinner table.

Whether the positive or the negative view is the one that works best for you, just be certain to try it whenever the urge to eat strikes you. Just flash the appropriate image into your mind. This should give you a few seconds to pause to consider whether what you're about to eat is something that will help or hinder your diet.

Come close to the glass

Next time you look in a mirror in private, stick your face right up next to the glass. You'll notice that your image is slightly blurred, or doubled, like a television "ghost" image. That's because most mirrors are silvered surfaces under a sheet of clear glass. The ghost image is your reflection on the surface of the glass, while your "real" reflection is on the silver behind the glass. Put your fingernail on your mirror and you'll see that it doesn't quite touch the reflected image on the silver surface.

I think it's important to understand a little about the properties of mirrors since you'll be relying on them for an important part of your life. But more important is your understanding of the imperfections of mirrors. Since you're not getting a true image of yourself in any mirror, being aware of it can help you compensate for the imperfections.

As for the ghost image in most mirrors, you probably cannot do much about it. There are such things as front-surfaced mirrors, which as the name describes, have the silver reflective surface uncovered. These mirrors are optically much purer than regular mirrors. Consequently, they are used for scientific purposes. Unfortunately, they are too delicate and breakable for everyday use. Just keep in mind that the mirrors you normally use won't be giving you the whole, crystal-clear picture. Which is one more reason why you should look into them so often—the more visual information you can gather about your own image, the better, so keep looking into the mirror.

Fun house mirrors

When the mirror method was first presented to a large group of people, one young lady asked about the distorting mirrors you sometimes see in carnival sideshows. By distorting the silver reflective surface of a mirror, you get a distorted reflection. That's how you can see a reflection of yourself stretched out to about nine feet tall or scrunched down to a mushroom with feet.

One enterprising local manufacturer of mirrors set up a retail store in a posh neighborhood. It featured good quality mirrors in expensive frames. The centerpiece of every display was a specially designed mirror in a frame slightly larger than on all the others in the grouping. The frame contained a mirror with just a hint of the fun house distortion effect—the one that makes you appear taller and thinner. This store sold many more of the special mirrors than of any other kind. The frame holding the special mirror cost approximately twenty-five dollars more than the other frames. The mirror itself cost only a few dollars more than the normal mirrors. But the price tag on each of these mirrors was marked up 100 percent over the price of any other mirror in the shop.

Don't be fooled by your mirror image

If you find a mirror that makes you look better than most other mirrors, do not purchase it. Do, however, buy the highest quality mirror you can afford. The higher the quality, the fewer imperfections in the reflective surface. There are enough strange things going on in even the best mirrors without you adding anything to the problem.

Your mirror image is a reverse image. In order to see yourself as others see you, it is necessary to place two mirrors side by side at a 90-degree angle (not necessarily an exact 90 degrees—you can move one mirror through different angles to change your view of yourself). It helps to mount a mirror on a wall next to another mirror that is on hinges (on a door, perhaps, like the mirrors on medicine cabinets). That way, you can adjust the hinged mirror to get a true picture of your face, profile, and back of your head.

If you can get two large mirrors to be mounted in the same manner as above, do so. In any case, even if you have to hold a hand mirror out to the side of another mirror, you'll be amazed at how different you look. You're used to seeing yourself in a reversed format, and some of your physical imperfections tend not to be noticed when you see yourself the same incorrect way day after day. Seeing yourself correctly, as others see you, may be a shock. You'll notice if you have some scowl marks, if you carry one shoulder lower than the other (I do), have a stooped posture, too much weight in one portion of your body, and so forth. Getting the real view of yourself should be a refreshing change after the initial shock wears off. It's a change in perspective that's a healthy part of the mirror method.

By the way, if you can get three mirrors mounted together, you'll be able to duplicate the "hall of infinite mirrors" effect like in the end of *Citizen Kane*.

Look at the shape of your face

One thing many people fail to notice is that their face is not symmetrical. That is, the left half of your face is not the same as the right side of your face.

This is a bit hard to prove to some people, but it can be done. You need to take two photos of your face, both the same size and both from the same straight-on angle. First, take one by aiming the camera into a mirror (get a friend to hold the camera; if you take your own picture you'll have to "shoot from the hip" or from your chest so as not to hide your face). Second, have someone take a "normal" portrait-type photo, being careful to match the same angle as the image taken in the mirror. Watch your sizing of the image of your face. It's deceptive because the distance from the camera to your face is not the same as it looks when you're shooting your mirror image. You have to combine the distance from you to the mirror and from the mirror to the camera.

Don't worry if both photos look like bad passport photos. A high-quality image isn't the point. Instant cameras are quite good for this job because you can check to see if you have your face the same size in each setup.

Once you have the two photographs of yourself, one being your mirror image and the other being your true image, cut them in two from top to bottom with the cut line running down your nose. Tape the right half of the photo taken of your mirror image to the left half of the other, conventional, photo and, presto—a weird picture of your face. You'll see that no matter whether you double the left or right side of your face, the resulting symmetrical photo does not look quite right.

The point of all this is to get you to really examine yourself. You've had years and years of being fooled by mirrors, so you need to look into them and at yourself in new ways in order to get a correct view of yourself. Further, looking into the mirror is a good way to remind yourself of your own importance and of your commitment to The Ego Diet.

Another oddity you should realize about mirrors is that they only show your image one-half normal size. This is easy to prove. Take a ruler and hold it up against a mirror. At arm's length, measure your head's reflection from ear to ear. It will be somewhere around three and a half inches. Then hold the ruler up against your nose, lining up one end with the reflection of one ear. You'll see that your other ear lines up with the ruler about seven inches or so down the length of the ruler. If you don't have a ruler, just wait until the next time you steam up your bathroom mirror after taking a shower; stand at arm's length from the mirror and trace the reflection of your head by running a finger through the condensation on the mirror. Measure the width of the mirror image by holding up a straight edge like a pencil or piece of paper, then compare that to the actual width of your head.

Get the "big picture"

To compensate for the odd half-size effect of regular mirrors, get a magnifying mirror to glance into once in a while. This helps you study your skin. Besides, you'll be amazed at your body's appearance up close. Pores look very large, for example, and your entire face appears ravaged by some infernal machine. You might think you look so alarming in the magnifying mirror that you'll be really pleased about yourself when you go back to the normal mirror. This should give you an extra boost of confidence. After all, nobody ever sees you up close like in the magnifying mirror (it brings you "closer" to your skin than a kissing partner), so if you glance into it just before leaving the house in the morning, and then quickly glance into your regular mirror, you may feel much better about your looks. And that feeling is exactly the way you want to feel all day long: bright, confident, alert.

If you can make yourself feel better, you'll actually look better, too. Think about the people you know who are truly beautiful. Not images of people on billboards, or in the movies—I'm talking about people you know personally. Beauty comes not from weight or proportion or perfect teeth—it comes from inside you. Warm, vibrant, happy people are beautiful; spiteful, vindictive, whiners are not, no matter what their bodies look like. You've seen silver-haired grandmothers who are beautiful because they radiate a glow of goodness. And you've seen young, slim, women with good bodies who are complete bitches—and their physical charms go for naught.

You've met people who are cheerful. They actually look better than others you may know who possess nicer noses, better bodies, leaner limbs, and so on. The truly beautiful people are the ones with the beautiful attitude.

Obviously, your goal should be to get your body into its best shape possible, but your mental set can help the way you look along the way.

Getting yourself to feel happy and confident with the magnifying-mirror-then-the-normal-mirror routine is similar to a baseball player swinging a weighted bat before taking his regular, lighter-weight bat up to the plate. Or a basketball team working out in heavy shoes prior to a game . . . they seem so much lighter when they switch to the lightweight tennies, they seem to float. You can do this mentally.

A middle-aged man who was a production line supervisor asked me about smiling on the job. "How can I maintain discipline among my employees when I go around with a big grin on my puss all the time?" Well, first of all, you don't have to smile all the time, but the primary thing to remember is this: if you're normally a fellow with an easy smile, just imagine how much more effective your disapproval will be when it must be meted out to an employee. Your workers will work harder to earn your constant smile while avoiding your frown.

Don't worry about age lines

Some people have tried the magnifying mirror routine and complained that they see their age lines, worry wrinkles, laugh lines, and so forth. This they find disconcerting. Unless you're not keeping your face clean or letting it get too dry and cracked, don't worry about age lines. Consider something Yves Montand, the French singer and film star once said about youth, appearance, and mental outlook: "Staying young in your life has nothing to do with trying to stay young in your face." In other words, don't try to hide your age or disguise your physical appearance. You are who you are—the most important person in the world—and the way you look is . . . perfect! The Ego Diet is just here to help you fully realize your perfection and then maintain it.

Certainly you should try to be well groomed and appropriately dressed, but good looks are really created in your heart and in your soul, not with broadcloth and blusher.

Use a camera along with your mirrors

With a little practice you should be able to take photos of yourself for study purposes. Take photos of yourself, nude and dressed, from as many angles as you can and look at them critically for proper posture, weight, clothing, and overall appearance.

You might want to get really dressed up for one of these sessions. But you should consider taking a few shots of yourself when you're really grungy. You don't have to go out in public like that, but it does you good to get down and dirty every now and again. As for how you should dress when going out, you can use this as a guide: dress the way you'd most like to be photographed by the press. That should keep you looking nice as well as dressed appropriately for the occasion.

When you are taking photos of yourself in the nude, you might be tempted to strike some poses. Women are fond of imitating models in *Playboy* or of dancing. You'll find that the poses in *Playboy* have very little to do with any kind of movement. The reason for this was best described in a line of a review of the nude musical *Oh Calcutta!* "The trouble with nude dancing," the reviewer wrote, "is that not everything stops when the music does."

You can ignore your scale

With the mirror method, you can decide to ignore your scale and simply concentrate on your image. You may indeed weigh more than some diet charts tell you to weigh, but if you look and feel great, that's all that counts.

On the other hand, if you are so completely conditioned to checking your pounds on a scale, fine. The one thing you don't want to do is stop your Ego Diet procedures after losing just a couple of pounds. Some people get so proud of the first few pounds they shed that they forget to remain on their diet. Meanwhile, as they're telling everyone they know about those two missing pounds, three new pounds are being added to their waistline.

You shouldn't have any trouble checking yourself out in mirrors. It's fun to do. And for some reason, mirrors have always had a fascination for most people. Especially creative people. Look at how often mirrors are used in books and films. In *Orphee,* a large mirror became the liquid door to another world. In *Alice Through the Looking Glass,* the mirror was also entrance to a whole world of fantasy. *Dracula* and *Nosferatu*—and the countless other vampire stories after them—showed us how a dead soul casts no reflection. In *The Gorgon,* you were turned to stone if you gazed upon the monster but were safe if you viewed it in a mirror. Remember the magic mirror in *Snow White?* Or the evil mirror in *Dead of Night?* Or the shootout sequence in Orson Welles's *Lady from Shanghai?* There are many other examples.

When you see a mirror, smile. You've got a secret way to gain confidence and lose weight.

Smiling is good exercise

Keep smiling. It's better exercise than frowning. Smiling actually requires more muscles than frowning, and it tends to pull your facial skin in such a way as to combat gravity's pull.

Not only will you feel better by smiling—not only will your feeling better help you stay on your diet—but a couple of other good things will happen. You'll find that your friends will want to share your good feelings with you. You'll make more new friends, too.

One other thing: your enemies will stew in their own juices wondering what the hell you're up to.

4

Thinking Yourself Thin

YOUR mind is the strongest part of your body.

Of the 10 billion nerve cells in your body, most are in your brain. You may have upwards of 100 million nerve cells in only one cubic inch of your brain.

Every one of your nerve cells, or neurons, communicates information. You are a mass of electronic information processing, because the neurons transmit signals through electric current.

At the same time, the brain is operating chemically. In reality, each of us is like a walking science laboratory combined with a power generating plant and a telephone switching company. And, since pure information signals are being sent through your nerves to all parts of your body—and reactions to these signals as well as reactions to the world outside your body are being sent back to your brain—you're somewhat like an incredibly swift, highly sophisticated, and extremely temperamental computer.

The control center of your body is in your mind. At any given second, one neuron in your brain may be communicating with up to 250,000 neighboring neurons. They, in turn, send signals on to other neurons, and so on throughout your body. The entire enterprise is incredibly complex, and . . . beautiful. Such wonderful design work seems to have gone into the creation of the human brain and body.

There is even a communication network between the left and right sides of your brain. Information received by one hemisphere of your brain is transferred over to the other hemisphere. While you're moving through your life, nerves are receiving sensory impulses and sending motor impulses (that is, commands for your body to perform some task, like blink, lift your arm, and so on). The spinal cord and brain together form a central nervous system and act as a kind of "automatic brain." If you touch something that is hot, you'll jerk your hand away before the realization of the heat fully sinks into your consciousness. Your nervous system simply did its job and reacted automatically.

However, you are in control of many other activities. Although your neurons, nerves, brain, central nervous system, peripheral nervous system, and muscles all "talk" to one another in every move you make, the fact is that you can decide to walk to the couch, stretch, sit, stand back up, walk to the refrigerator, open it, and decide to have . . . cookies or a piece of fruit.

And that's where The Ego Diet enters the picture.

Your imagination

Human beings may not be the only animals capable of imagining things, but it is certainly true that this ability is an attribute of creatures with higher intelligence. With your imagination, you can create anything. Sights you've never seen can become complete, panoramic vistas in your mind's eye. Sounds you've never heard can float in and out of your inner ear.

You can build mental pictures of people, places, and things. You can change these pictures at will, and that's important because you may not have a good mental picture of yourself. You can take some steps to change that.

Describe yourself—in perspective

Think about how you think about yourself. Be honest. Be as forthright as you can be—as if you were confiding in a doctor willing to devote a long time to your case.

Many people who are overweight have depressing images of themselves. Time after time, people take me aside and whisper their upsetting self-images to me. They say they put on a strong false front when dealing with others, but they really feel angry, hurt, sad, or even ashamed of their bodies. Which is a shame because it represents wasted energy.

There is no need to feel enraged at yourself because you're a few pounds—or even many pounds—overweight. Nor is there any need to get angry over the fact that you've tried and failed on a diet plan. It's not the end of the universe, after all, and you're now taking the right steps to clear up the situation.

A lack of self-esteem seems to hit women particularly hard, probably because women are judged by the look of their bodies more often and more harshly than are men. This is grossly unfair, but our society doesn't seem to be moving rapidly to change this state of affairs, so you'll just have to live with it. The negative self-view isn't limited to women, but it strikes them unusually hard, so hard that some women even seem to deny their good features. It may seem odd that some smart, successful, talented, and otherwise beautiful women can downgrade all that to the point of emotional breakdown just because of some extra pounds.

The lesson to be learned here is that it's not unheard of to be terribly down on yourself over your weight, but that everything must be viewed in its proper perspective. You make value judgments about others as well as yourself: some are conscious; some are in your unconscious mind. But all of them cannot help but be influenced by the value judgments others make, especially those made by people with media clout (the people who make movies, TV shows, and advertisements). What are we supposed to think when gorgeous, svelte, and perfectly proportioned people stare back at us from magazines, billboards, TV screens, and motion picture screens? Not only are most stars quite easy on the eyes, there are many highly trained (and highly paid) individuals responsible for their hair, make-up (yes, on the male stars, too), wardrobe, dialogue, lighting, and choreography or poses. Everything can be made perfect for a movie or an ad. Even if someone isn't perfect in an ad (as I wasn't), the ad agency usually planned it that way.

In any event, there are far more images of perfection out there than there are images of reality. (The nightly news is one notable exception. Somehow, this dose of the harsh realities of life in no way compensates for the deluge of unrealistic "prettified" people in the media.)

Just because the make-up man, lighting director, cameraman, wardrobe designer, and director have managed to hide any blemishes, bulges, or blotches on the actors and actresses you see in ads and films is no reason to get upset. These people are in the business of selling fantasy, so it is their job to make everything look great. It's fun. It's a form of escape. And it's very attractive. But it ain't real, folks, and you shouldn't compare yourself to this celluloid dream state.

Compare yourself to yourself

Instead of worrying that you don't look as good as the models in the clothing commercials, try thinking you are as trim as you'd like to be. If you want to get really elaborate, imagine yourself in those commercials. But no fair imagining yourself ten years younger or with a full head of hair if you don't have one now. Also no fair imagining yourself six inches taller than you are. (You can gain an inch of height with proper posture, as you saw in Chapter 3, but that's it.)

You might wonder why I took the time to set up an understanding of the mind and brain, only to tell you not to fully exercise your powers of imagination. What I'm really trying to prevent is your falling under the spell of those unrealistic images presented by the media. If you don't have the same age, height, body structure, hair, and so on as your favorite movie star role model, then what's the point of imagining that you do? You're just going to depress your spirits even further in the long run.

Instead, use your imagination in a healthy manner. Take what you've been given to work with, and build from there. For heaven's sake, it's enough of a triumph to imagine yourself as you truly can be in just a few weeks. You don't have to clutter up things with a media-induced fantasy.

Get a mental picture of yourself as you'd like to be in six weeks. Remember, you're the same height, same age, and same body structure, but you can imagine yourself at your ideal weight, with properly fitting clothes, and with a feeling of self-satisfaction and inner grace. You can imagine yourself with a deep, peaceful contentment. You can imagine yourself being admired by others.

All right, now: Compare this image with the way you are at this moment. Before you get depressed about the difference, simply ask yourself this one logical—but often overlooked—question: Is there anything you can do right now that will bring you a little closer to your imagined self? Did you imagine yourself wearing certain colors of clothing? You can wear similar colors now. Just because you weigh more now and will weigh less in a few weeks doesn't change the fact that you should design your wardrobe around the seasonal colors that are right for you.

Did you imagine yourself with a good hairstyle? Well, nothing is preventing you from getting that style right now. Just because you weigh more now has nothing to do with the style of hair that suits your head shape. True, your face will be thinner in a few weeks, but your head will still have the same overall appearance, so your hairstyle should work at any weight.

There are undoubtedly several other small things you can do at this moment to bring you immediately closer to your ideal self. Don't wait until later on to do them . . . you're already on The Ego Diet, so get moving with the most enjoyable parts of it!

Another good reason for comparing

Think of your imagined self, your ideal image. Got it? Good. This time, instead of comparing that perfected image to the way you are right now, compare your ideal image to the way you might be when you're halfway between then and now.

If you're trying to lose fifty pounds, you can easily see yourself thinner and you can easily see yourself as you are now, but it's sometimes difficult to imagine yourself just twenty-five pounds slimmer (unless you remember yourself when you *were* twenty-five pounds slimmer). Still, it'll be worth it to make the effort.

Okay, now split the difference once again. Imagine how you'll look after having lost twelve and a half pounds. Now perform this imaginary weight gain once more. How will you look after losing about six pounds? Three pounds? How about a pound and a half? Consider the difference between weighing what you weigh right now and what you'll be like after losing half a pound.

Now you have the way you're going to look after one day on The Ego Diet. Certainly you can lose *more* than a half a pound your first day on the diet, but why bother? You already know where you're going to end up. You already know what you'll look like at every step along the way. You already know that getting there takes time. So resolve right now to do just enough of The Ego Diet to lose one-half pound tomorrow.

A case history

I worked in an office with a young man I'll call David. He was an amazingly bright person, eager to learn, and possessed of the kind of good manners one associates with old movies and the Senate dining room. David had come to this country from Cuba when he was quite young, and although he spoke our language beautifully (better than several native Americans in the office, to be truthful about it), he did have a slight, lilting accent.

David was—and is—a poet. He was only working in our office to earn enough money to write and attempt to get published. He also was fond of traveling around town to various gatherings of other poets where he would wait his turn to get up and recite his work.

His poems were full of strange juxtapositions of beauty and violence, reflecting his sensibilities—he was vibrantly, lovingly aware of the joys of life, yet constantly shocked at the unfairness and ugliness that is also found in the world. Having come to English as a second language, he often used words in new and unusual contexts in his poems. While some of us found this both charming and distracting, many of his peers were unreservedly pleased to read his work and/or hear him speak.

It is in this latter area that David came to need the help of The Ego Diet.

If you get up in front of people

You can imagine the fears you'd have if you were about to face a group of poetry lovers, critics, and fellow writers with your newest work. You know what it's like to speak in front of a group of people. Your stomach tightens up. Your palms get sweaty. Your legs feel like gelatin. And that's just the night before the speech.

Everyone feels like this. The famous actor who has appeared in two hundred and fifty stage plays feels just as nervous as the guy at the backyard party who is suddenly put on the spot when someone in a big booming voice says "Tell us all about that fence you're going to put up to keep our kids and our dogs off your creeping bent!" The well-known nightclub comedian who makes his living going on stage twice a night to improvize his show is just as nervous as the gal who is chosen to make a presentation to her fellow office workers about the new pension plan. The celebrated after-dinner speaker who gets a great deal of money just to deliver a set speech is just as nervous as any student who is called on to recite in the classroom. We all get nervous. If we didn't, the adrenaline wouldn't start flowing inside us and there would be no spark, no excitement in anything we said when "on stage." Adrenaline is a hormone that your body secretes during any fearful situation. It stimulates you; artificial forms of adrenaline may be used as a heart stimulant.

David was no different when it came to speaking in front of people. He got nervous, but the joy of being able to present a piece of his art—his poetry—was stronger than his fear of getting up in front of the crowd . . . until he began gaining weight.

Weight and worry

It's a funny thing about getting a little older, but you can go along only so far in life eating a certain amount of rich or junky foods without having any trouble with excess flab. But as soon as you reach a particular age—in David's case around twenty-five years old—your body doesn't assimilate the food in the same manner as when you were a few years younger. You can get a potbelly before you even know it.

That's what happened to David. He was basically a thin, lithe person, yet here he was changing day by day until his shadow began to resemble a match stick with a blob of jelly in the middle. When he noticed his extra weight, he began to worry about it. Worrying caused him to nibble more snacks between meals. Snacking caused him to gain more weight. Which made him worry more. He got so caught up in his very minor weight problem that he was afraid to go read his poetry in public. "I can't go up in front of those people looking like this," he once muttered to me. I don't think that was the entire problem.

He was actually feeling less worthy as a person and as an artist because he couldn't seem to control his body, and this self-deprecation was causing him to question whether he was able to create. This unrealistically harsh critical attitude *was* affecting his work. "I'm not writing as much as before," he complained. "And what I write isn't too good lately. I don't know what it is," he sighed. This just gave him even more to worry about, leading to another vicious circle of overeating and self-deprecation.

I thought I knew what part of his problem was, but I couldn't just come right out and say it. Or at least I couldn't think of a polite way to do so at that time. Today, I might feel differently because of my discovering a side benefit of having written The Ego Diet—the benefit grew out of the countless discussions I had about this diet plan, discussions with people from almost every walk of life. Eventually, I found that it's much easier to swing the subject of dieting into the conversation if you begin on another topic—like a discussion of the power of the human ego, for example.

The confession

After going along in a depressed state for several weeks, David finally made up his mind to talk about his situation. He waited until most people had left the building. Even so, he still made certain to take me aside so we would be speaking in a private office. His tone as he began was muted. We were conversing almost conspiratorially, as if we were plotting some sort of dastardly act.

Finally, he got to the point:

"What, um, do you do to stay thin?" he asked. "I mean," he added, "you seem to eat stuff all the time but you never gain weight."

Like almost everyone with whom I've worked, he noticed that I like to eat lunch from about ten in the morning until just before five in the afternoon. The secret is that I never do it on days when I go out for a normal, full-sized luncheon meal. If I bring my lunch to work, I enjoy starting on it early and finishing it late, saving the sandwich for the traditional noon lunch hour. So although it might look like I'm consuming more food than most people, it's not really the case at all.

It turned out that David was not only worried about his protruding tummy, his lack of concentration while trying to write, his lack of quality output, and his overall worth as a writer, he was also caught up in a comparison with other people. In this case, he was unfairly comparing himself with the images on movie screens as well as someone he knew, namely me.

"How do you do it?" he pleaded, "how do you keep from gaining weight?"

I had an instant of confusion as the mass of data that is now this book swam in front of my head, and then I blurted out two short, cryptic words: "Think thin," was all I said. But I said it very authoritatively.

David got one of those "gosh I hope I'm not dealing with a maniac" looks on his face as he slowly mouthed my two mysterious words.

I could understand his plight. Here he'd been belaboring this question in his mind for days, only to find, once he'd got up enough courage to ask it, that "think thin" was his only guideline. It was a perfect example of the old joke about the man spending months struggling through the wilds and climbing mountains in order to find a hermit holy man and ask him "What is the meaning of life?"—and then getting an answer that's as substantial as raw pabulum, something like "Life is a cup of chewing gum, my son." [The rest of the joke, for those of you who haven't experienced it, is simply this: The young man, stunned, shouts angrily at the hermit, "I've sweated blood to get here only to find out you think the meaning of life is 'a cup of chewing gum'?" To which the hermit replies, surprised, "You mean it isn't?"]

"I want . . . I don't want . . .

I started over again with David. I asked him to tell me about his eating habits. After the usual items (he was comparatively very good about eating balanced meals), he got to what he perceived to be his problem area:

"It's the cookies," he said. "Well, anything sweet, really, but I keep eating cookies at home, sometimes right out of the bag. And then there's the sweet rolls and doughnuts here at work."

He paused, then added, "You know, it's funny, but I don't want to eat them. Not really. But I want to taste them. Oh I don't know . . . I want 'em but I don't want 'em. Isn't that weird?"

"Not at all," I said. "You see, if I understand what's happening to you and your eating habits, you're caught in something called an approach-avoidance conflict. That's where your desire for something is offset by something else that makes you turn away from it."

"You mean," he said, "like cookies and calories?"

"Right. You want the taste of the sugar, but you know the calories are going to hurt you, so you're caught in the middle. What's happening is that you're worrying about the approach-avoidance conflict. Or, rather, you're upset because you can't seem to resolve the conflict. But now that you know about it, it will be a little easier to deal with it."

"Well," he said, "I don't know . . ." He was dubious that simply knowing part of his problem had a name would help clear up the problem.

"Look," I said, "it's not as simple as that. You just need a different way to deal with your desire for sugar, your desire to eat, and your eating habits as a whole, and I think I've got the way."

How thinking thin works

I said to David, "You never really worried about eating cookies before you found yourself a little overweight, did you?"

"No, but I don't think I ate this many cookies before, either."

"Okay, but don't worry about that," I said, "Part of the reason you're eating more of them is that you're worried about eating them. You're eating to try to resolve a problem. Before, when you were at the weight you want to be, you'd sometimes have some sugar as a kind of reward to yourself. Or you'd have some sugar when you were annoyed about something, and the good taste of it seemed to make things better. Now, you're trying to get rid of an annoyance *and* you're trying to reward yourself for wanting to write. The trouble is, you aren't writing because you're annoyed at yourself because of your weight. And you're annoyed about your weight because of eating too many cookies, so—

"So it's a vicious circle," he concluded.

"You bet," I said. "But here's the point: As I said, you weren't having this problem back when you were a thin person, right?"

"Right . . ."

"All right. So you're a thin person. Now your problem is gone."

"What?" he said.

"Bear with me, now: if you think of yourself as a thin person, you won't have the problem of worrying about your weight. After all, a thin person doesn't have that particular worry. Also, you won't have the approach-avoidance conflict, because a thin person wouldn't go eat all those cookies."

He grinned and said, "Is this a variation on 'I think, therefore I am'?" He was referring to one of the famous quotes by the French metaphysical philosopher René Descartes (1596–1650), who said that mind and soul were as one, and proved his own existence by the following argument: "I doubt I exist; but who is doing the doubting? Therefore, *Cogito, ergo sum* (I think, therefore I am)."

So David found a new twist on Descartes. He asked, "Is it now 'I think I'm thin, therefore I'm thin'?"

"Sort of," I replied. "If you imagine yourself being the thin person you want to be, you'll approach every bit of food in a different manner. Don't think about your diet, think instead that you, a thin person, doesn't need to eat those fattening things. See, a thin person wouldn't eat all those cookies; therefore, you won't eat all those cookies. Use the power of your imagination to see yourself thin. You can do it. Your mind is amazingly strong."

I continued to describe the benefits of the thinking-thin method, particularly relating it to the ways his writing would be improved. Freed from the worry of weight, and not distracted by the need for constant "rewards" of sugar, he would be a new man. He would be the important poet he knew he was. And, in a very short time, he would be as thin as he imagined himself to be.

I also pointed out that he, as a person in the arts, was especially suited to the thinking-thin method because it involved the imagination. Artists are often called right-brain people—people who like the more abstract disciplines such as music and art. Left-brain people, who are more analytical and who therefore feel more comfortable with numbers and symbols, are just as likely to have success with the thinking-thin method of The Ego Diet, but their response to it rests more on the psychological sense of it. In other words, they react better to the reasoning behind the method—the explanation and directions—than to the idea of using the power of their imaginations. Either type of person has the ability to use the mind-over-matter technique in the thinking-thin method; they just approach it from opposite sides.

At this point in our conversation, David broke in with a question that suddenly popped into his head:

"What if I am reaching for some cookies not because I'm trying to get the sugar but because I'm really hungry?"

"Well," I said, "would a thin person reach for cookies if he was 'really hungry,' as you put it?"

"I guess not," he admitted sheepishly.

"Right. A thin person like you would convert the craving for cookies into a craving for something healthy. Imagine how a great, fresh salad with all sorts of meats, cheeses, and sliced lettuce tastes. Imagine how a big, lusciously plump and juicy orange tastes—with the drops of sun-yellow liquid flowing across your tongue!" I was getting into this. David didn't mind. He was joining in:

"How about a ripe pineapple?" he asked. "Those taste great! And really good tomatoes! Where can I get some good ones?"

I suggested a couple of small groceries that were known for having fresh produce. It turned out that one of them was part of a small chain of specialty markets and there was one in his neighborhood. We're not all that fortunate, but good foods are available out there if you look for them.

Act like the thin person you want to be

You know what's realistic for you. If you have no doubt about your being able to wear a certain size swimsuit or a certain tight cut of sports clothing (or whatever you set your hopes on), then imagine yourself in that outfit. Acting like the thin person you are going to be will help you get there faster.

You might have to practice thinking yourself thin. You will do better if you can make it a habit.

It's a matter of getting the message firmly into the association areas of your brain—those parts of the brain with extremely complex connections between neurons. The association areas are thought to produce our more complicated thinking patterns, actions, and feelings.

David obviously did it—he lost weight, went back on his "lecture circuit," continued writing, and his first book of poems was published just four months prior to my writing this chapter. If David can do it and I can do it, so can you.

5

In A Pinch

YOU don't need charts and graphs to tell you if you're overweight. You don't even need scales.

Here's why. No matter what method of weight-to-height ratio is used, all weight charts have a basic, built-in flaw: they all rely on somebody's definition of "normal body weight."

Name a method of finding your proper weight—it has that same flaw. It doesn't matter whether you go by body water content or body density (weight per unit of volume—this is the one that attempts to adjust the weight charts to compensate for whether you're big-boned or possessed of a small frame). It doesn't matter if your source is big or small, famous or unknown, every chart must take into consideration someone's subjective view.

This is not to say that body weight is all just a matter of opinion. It's not. There *are* some charts and graphs that are quite valid and medically sound. These are the actuarial tables compiled by insurance companies. They spend a great amount of time and effort to update and maintain these tables because their business depends on them.

An actuarial table is prepared by a team of statisticians who work with large numbers of events—events such as deaths, for instance. Since life insurance claims are the only certainty in the insurance game, it is crucial for the companies to know the odds for and against your death at any given age. But they cannot stop there. They must gather hundreds and thousands of facts to correlate with the two basic facts of age and sex. With the aid of computers, it is possible for the insurance companies to figure the odds on the likelihood of death for a member of either sex at any age as it relates to:

smoking
exercise
childhood diseases

parental diseases
occupation
drinking
driving
travel
residence
number of miles traveling to work
weight-to-height ratio

It is this gathering of information that is respectable. When insurance companies decide to publish some of their tables, you can be fairly certain that the information is as accurate as it can be, for a great deal of money is riding on their predictions. So if their tables say you're over-weight by eight pounds, I'd tend to string along with their assessment.

Still, the fact is that you don't even need the insurance company actuarial tables to know if you're overweight. You can tell by pinching yourself.

Pinching yourself?

Yes, You'll see how it can be done in a few minutes. First, it might be a good idea to discuss what it is about your body that allows the pinch procedure to work.

Even thin people have fat

Based on actuarial studies, there are two different percentages of fat that are considered ideal for the human body. If you're a man, your body functions best with about 12 to 15 percent fat (assuming fairly normal physical activity: people in jobs requiring bulk and brawn, like football players, may have different needs; people in jobs requiring speed, like runners, have different needs again). If you're a woman, your body functions best with about 22 to 25 percent fat (again, assuming reasonably normal physical activity).

So even if you're a few pounds overweight, you can be happy about the fact that even your thin friends have as much as 25 percent body fat. Another way of looking at this, and a more positive way, is that you don't have to lose all the fat on your body. You only have to get down to 15 or 25 percent.

Where is the body fat?

Well, that depends on the body. Seriously, most body fat is found in one part of your body—the area just below the surface of your skin.

Because about half of the total fat lies immediately under the skin, you can keep tabs on it by gently but firmly pinching yourself. You just have to know how to do it. Yes, I'm saying you don't know how to pinch. In this case, there is a trick to it.

Before we get to the pinch procedure, you should know that it doesn't have the accuracy of a method that has a more scientific history, a method used to weigh battleships!

There is a perfectly precise way to measure your own percentage of body fat, but it is not at all practical for most of us. Still, for those of you who desire to know your exact body fat percentage, here is the water displacement method and how it works: At a clinic, university, or private fitness center that is properly equipped for the test, your body can be weighed while it is displacing water from a tank. What you weigh when in water, compared to the weight of the water that is displaced (or spilled over the edge of the tank—the tank having been filled to the rim before you enter), is proportional to the muscle-to-fat ratio in your body.

The pinch procedure will not give as precise a measurement as the water displacement method, but you can see why trying the latter method in your bathtub wouldn't be a good idea. Unless, of course, you happen to like wet floors.

The pinch procedure

You can use your finger and thumb as calipers to measure the body fat you have at various parts of your body. By comparing the results of the procedure from two specific portions of your body you can estimate your body's percentage of body fat.

To get used to the way the pinch should be performed, grab a fold of skin above your lowest rib straight down from your shoulder. Take care to check if you are grabbing skin plus the layer of fat that lies beneath; there is another layer below the layer of body fat—a layer of muscle. The muscle layer is tougher and is therefore fairly easily separated from the layer of fat.

You might want to try pinching yourself several times, each time separating the underlying muscle layer. The idea is to get used to telling the difference while at the same time not letting your thumb and finger work their way out to the edge of the skin fold.

Once you're accustomed to grasping a large area of skin and separating fat from muscle, you're ready to begin your pinch procedure.

Press the skin fold together and measure to the nearest quarter of an inch. With your free hand, hold a ruler next to your thumb and finger to check the distance they are apart.

Repeat the procedure in the same general area to improve your accuracy. Get someone to perform the measurements on you as a check to see if you're both doing it properly.

There are two areas of the body, other than the area near your ribs, that are particularly well suited to this measurement. Both men and women can pinch the middle of the front of the thigh, making certain that the skin fold is perpendicular to the ground. In other words, the fold should run up and down in a straight line with your leg. This test should be performed while standing. The second test for men involves the abdomen. Again, while standing, pinch yourself just to the side of your navel with the fold running parallel to the ground. The second test for women uses the upper part of the arm. While sitting or standing, pinch the middle of the back part of your arm, between your shoulder and elbow. The fold should run perpendicular to the floor.

Now, if you wish to include the measurements from your rib along with these two other places, you'll have three different numbers you can use.

What do these numbers mean?

The rib measurement is the least accurate but the easiest to monitor on a daily basis. You can even perform it during the day to remind yourself not to eat the wrong foods. Basically, if you find over an inch between your finger and thumb on the rib pinch, you have excessive body fat to diet away. If you have just under an inch, you could stand to lose a few pounds. If you have a half inch, you're doing extremely well and probably just need to maintain your current diet.

Bear in mind that you must relate what you feel in the pinch procedure to what you see in the mirror. If you don't like your shape, take a pinch and remember what the pinch feels like at this stage of your life. Then, as you pinch yourself to keep reminding yourself to avoid the overeating, you'll be able to chart your progress in your own hand, so to speak.

The thigh and abdomen tests (for men) and the thigh and arm tests (for women) should be examined together. For men, you are at your ideal percentage of fat if your thigh measurements are in the following relation to your abdomen measurements:

thigh	abdomen
(all measurements in inches)	
3	¼
2¾	¼
2½	¼
2¼	¼–½
2	½
1¾	½–¾
1½	½–¾
1¼	¾
1	¾–1
¾	1
½	1–1¼
¼	1–1¼

For women, you are at your ideal percentage of fat if your thigh measurements are in the following relation to your arm measurements:

thigh	arm
(all measurements in inches)	
2	½
1¾	½–¾
1½	½–1
1¼	¾–1¼
1	1–1½
¾	1¼–1¾
½	1½–2

Weight is somewhat relative

With the pinch procedure, you will be able to ignore the number of pounds you weigh in favor of how you look and (literally) how you feel. This is important for two reasons. First, since muscle weighs more than fat, a trim and muscled individual may weigh the same as a larger, flabby person. Second, an ideal weight is frequently a matter of opinion. Speaking as a man, I can state categorically that while there are many very sexy looking thin females in the world, there are many more very sexy looking average-weighing women around. There are even many enticing and sexy looking women who are what used to be called zaftig. It is only women who do not have any muscle tone—who have what can only be called flab on them—that are a turnoff to me. I'm certain that a glance in any of the current issues of *Playboy* will convince you that it is not only the thin gals who attract the guys.

The first problem with the pinch procedure

There are two pitfalls with the pinch procedure that you should know about.

The first is no big deal . . . unless you happen to be Italian.

There is a tradition in Italy that men are allowed to pinch women when in public. True, this phenomenon has been played up by the media beyond its significance. And true, this tradition has been of late more honored in the breach than in the observance. Yet it does happen. Italian women are able to handle it (some say it's the Italian men who are truly able to handle it), but tourists are frequently taken aback.

When I was explaining the pinch procedure to a group of people, one Italian man spoke up in mild protest.

"You are, dare I say it? putting the finishing touches on a proud custom."

There is a scene in the comedy *Who Is Killing The Great Chefs of Europe?* (worth seeing for Robert Morley's performance and the extremely clever satirical comments about food) when Jacqueline Bisset is discussing one of the film's murders with an Italian man of good character. He has been very polite all through their talk, which takes place in an open-air market. They both pause to let Bissett squeeze some melons. A man passes behind her. She starts in alarm, whirls around on the man, tells him what she thinks of him, and he slinks off. Her male companion, again acting most politely, inquires about her reaction.

"That man pinched me!" she says, shocked.

"Oh no," he calmly assures her, "that was me."

After all, he did have to keep in practice.

The second problem with the pinch procedure

There is an unfortunate tendency among couples who are using the pinch procedure to perform a different kind of pinching on each other. While some of this activity is done in a playful manner, I have found that it can easily escalate to an annoying level.

Particularly upsetting is the sort of pinching accompanied by teasing that mocks the person who is seeking to control a diet. This is to be avoided because it undercuts the effectiveness of The Ego Diet. When you're working on deprogramming your own mind from its old patterns—patterns that made you eat too much, of the wrong foods, at the wrong times—then you need support and understanding, not joking around. Your ego is a serious matter, and you can have any doubters read this book. If they try to grasp the psychological precepts set down in this and other chapters, perhaps then they'll realize that The Ego Diet is no laughing matter.

In any event, don't pinch your spouse or posslq (Person of Opposite Sex Sharing Living Quarters) except lovingly.

Make the pinching a habit

If the pinch procedure appeals to you and makes you comfortable, then you can use it to remind yourself to stay on track toward diet control.

When you think of food you shouldn't eat, pinch yourself. When you sit down for a meal, pinch yourself. When you consider having seconds, pinch yourself. When you think about dessert, pinch yourself.

Make it a habit and you'll find you'll always think twice about overeating, snacking, or indulging in rich, nonhealthful foods.

6

Make A List

YOU were on your first diet before you were born. Your mother fed you from within her body when you were an embryo, when you were a fetus, and right up to the moment of your birth.

There are no doubt many influences you carry with you from this period: why you like certain foods, why you dislike others, why you have a tendency to overeat at certain times and not others. This theory has been written about and discussed for many years but is as yet unproved.

What has been proved is the connection between your feeding/eating patterns as an infant and your eating habits now. Your early meals, which consisted of baby formula and/or mother's milk, were physical and psychological satisfiers. You were scared when your belly craved food, and you were satisfied with the bottle or nipple.

Gradually you were introduced to soft foods. Sometimes this was satisfying; other times, you wanted to return to the safe feeling you had with milk. This conflict, coupled with your parents' desire to set up scheduled, regular eating periods, led to forced feeding. They wanted you to eat when they ate, not when you wanted to eat. This led to more conflict about food. It was still a satisfier, but now it was a bit more difficult to obtain a fully peaceful satisfying meal.

In their efforts to get you to eat what they wanted you to eat, when they wanted you to eat it, your parents gradually introduced you to reward feeding. That is, you were rewarded with some foods you enjoyed if you ate some foods you didn't enjoy. In addition, you were rewarded for being quiet when your parents wanted peace; for not putting up a fuss during meals; for any number of seemingly insignificant things. But with each of these minor acts, you came to regard food as either a reward or a punishment.

You also gradually began to associate some foods with medicine. You were constantly urged to eat certain things because they would "make you grow big and strong" or because they would "help you stay well."

There was often a conflict between what you thought had a good taste and what your parents, relatives, baby-sitters, or neighbors felt was "good for you." Just as often, there was also a conflict over how much food you wanted to eat and the amount they wanted you to consume. Sometimes you got too much food; sometimes too little. And sometimes you got the opportunity to overeat with foods you liked. In this way you associated that satisfied feeling with overeating.

The media

As you were growing up, images of food and attitudes about food were promulgated by advertising, TV, and films. Of all the influences, advertising may have been the strongest. You hummed and sang commercial jingles about foods. You asked your parents for certain products you saw advertised. You memorized advertising slogans for food products.

What was being advertised?

Think about the foods that are advertised now. By and large, the same types of foods were advertised when you were growing up. The names of the products might have changed but the types of products remain all too similar.

Candy is heavily advertised, and primarily to children. There are some candy ads directed toward adults, but they are the exception rather than the rule.

Breakfast foods—cereals, instant "tarts," instant waffles, instant pancakes, and the like—are heavily advertised. These are more heavily advertised for children than they are for adults, but the number of ads directed at all age groups is higher than for candy because the makers of these products know they can hook you two ways: children like the promise of a sweet taste; adults like the idea of convenience. A breakfast food that can be quickly and easily prepared is one that can be delegated to the children. Thus you learned to feed yourself some sweets before the day was really started.

In this area of convenience, there is a group of advertisers that includes some of the biggest purveyors to both children and adults: the makers of fast food. Sometimes we refer to it as junk food. We've become so used to the term junkfood that we now think of it as just one word in many contexts.

(The Robert Morley character in *Who Is Killing The Great Chefs of*

Europe? sardonically refers to American fastfood/junkfood as "fake food.")

There are ads for hamburgers, hot dogs, fried chicken, pizza, frozen pizza, tacos, fish 'n' chips, and still more hamburgers practically everywhere you look these days.

Ads showing people enjoying these fastfood/junkfood items beam down at you from billboards, out at you from television sets, over you from radios, up at you from magazines . . . everybody seems to be healthy, happy, and wonderfully thin in these ads. Yet all they seem to eat are fastfood/junkfood items with the occasional salad (which is more than offset by the special dessert fastfood/junkfood items).

In a sense, you're still being treated like a child in that others are telling you to "eat this—you'll like it." Or my favorite line from the cereal commercials: "part of this delicious breakfast," which is delivered just as a table full of cereal, fruit, and some form of protein is shown. Yeah, I'd say it's a "part" of that delicious breakfast. That wording is a requirement of the federal government. I know because, like a lot of writers, I frequently work my wordsmithing for the very same ad agencies responsible for helping convince you to eat more food. The reason admakers are forced to show a breakfast consisting of more than just the cereal and milk, as well as saying "part of this delicious breakfast," is simple: the cereal and milk isn't a nutritious breakfast. So the government won't allow an ad that is for a product aimed at children to mislead kids into thinking the cereal alone is enough for a good breakfast. (There are many such restrictions affecting the makers of television commercials. This is why so many commercials for certain types of products all seem to be saying the same thing. It also accounts for the fact that many ads are just downright boring.)

You've had people tell you what to eat, when to eat, and how much to eat for most of your life. You've had food used as a reward or punishment for most of your childhood. You've had food used as a medicine at some point during your childhood. Now, you're using food improperly, causing you to weigh more than you'd like. Is it any wonder this has happened? And we haven't even touched on such problems as tension (at work, at home, at school), which can greatly influence your eating.

Analyze your eating habits

You can do a bit of research on yourself and your eating habits, and, with a little help, you can be your own psychologist. You'll know more about why you eat what you eat after doing the exercises in this chapter. And you may be able to use both the knowledge of why you eat and the technique for finding out to help you lose weight and keep it off.

The list

Step one is harder than it sounds. You must list what you eat during the day. Think back on your last twenty-four hours.

Now write down what you consumed. You probably had three regular meals. Each meal consisted of several things to eat and at least one beverage.

But what about between meals? Did you have some cookies, or candy, or crackers, or popcorn, or. . . .

The more you think about it, the longer your list becomes. "Oh yes, there was that cheese-and-crackers break. And a cup of tea—no, two cups." And so on.

Be honest. Put everything down on paper. Nobody has to see your list. You don't have to save the list if you don't want to do so. There will not be a torturous session of adding up the calories of everything on your list. All you need to do is get every bit of food you ate in one day listed on a piece of paper.

Okay. Think about this list of food items. You know which ones weren't so good for you and which ones were helpful. Do you realize that if you were to substitute one of the bad foods on your list for something good for you you'd start to lose weight? You can easily do that much, can't you? Of course you can. It's easy. Just take one thing —cookies and milk, perhaps, or the piece of pie after lunch—and trade it for a piece of fresh fruit or a fresh vegetable. There. You're on a new diet.

Make a new list the day after tomorrow and repeat the process. Yes, it is possible that you'll add some other new bad thing to your diet, but we'll see about removing that possibility in a minute.

Next time you think about eating something, think about adding it to your list. Will it look good on the list or will it make you cringe later on when you study it?

After you finish a meal and it's time for dessert, think about how much better your list will be without that dessert on it.

Before ordering a meal in a restaurant, think about how each menu item would look on your list. Will reading it make you happy or make you disappointed?

You can quickly arrive at the point where actually writing down your list becomes irrelevant—you'll be mentally composing your list all day long. This is the perfect means of behavior modification. You'll be reminding yourself to eat right without the psychological burden of telling yourself to stay on a diet. Instead, you'll be rewarding your own good behavior by giving yourself a "good grade" each time you add something healthy to your mental list. And you'll be happy every time you avoid a "wrong answer" by avoiding bad foods.

A mental list or a physical list?

For some reason, some people respond better to the mental list and others get a much better result if they do make a written list each day or every other day. Both methods work and both are psychologically valid. Both are part of The Ego Diet.

There seems to be no difference in the intellectual abilities of the people who write and the people who keep track mentally. At first I thought perhaps the mental list makers were smarter; then, since I write for a living, I assumed the pen-on-paper list makers were the smarter ones. But, as nearly as I can tell, there is no correlation between mental ability and the fact that some people like to keep the list in one form rather than another.

Whichever form you choose, just be certain you list all the foods or think about how every food will look on your list. And be certain to play fair with yourself by listing quantity. If you ate half a bag of salted toasted corn chips, then don't just put down "corn chips." If you had two cookies, list two cookies; if you had two dozen cookies, list two dozen cookies. The difference between a good, healthy diet and the poor diet that has caused you to gain weight may not have anything to do with what you eat—it may depend on the amount you eat.

You might be able to lose weight and maintain your ideal weight without changing your diet in any way except the size of your portions! You may be one of those lucky people who can still eat everything you've always eaten while on a lifelong diet. Try the list method for a week, altering only the amount of food you eat. Is there a difference in your weight? Do you look better? Do you feel better? If the answer is "yes" to any of these questions, The Ego Diet is already working for you.

Whether or not you can continue eating the same foods or must make a change, you still have the same problem all of us face: finding out why we eat the way we do.

Why . . .

Look over your list or review it in your mind. Is there anything obvious about your choice of foods? If you list everything in order (it helps to fill out the list as you go through the day), can you see a pattern in the way you eat?

For example, are you rewarding yourself with sweets when you eat your vegetables? Don't be ashamed to face up to this remnant of childhood behavior. I know this is the way I eat when I'm at work. I am careful to follow a sweet with an apple or tomato. I know this seems to be in reverse order for a reward, but I do it this way for a couple of reasons, and these reasons may also work for you.

First, I have come to associate the natural sugar in fruits with the artificial (in the sense of having too large an amount as well as being refined differently) sugar content of the cookies or brownies or whatever. Second, the good food helps clean my teeth after having the sweets.

Association of tastes

I find nothing wrong with rewarding yourself for eating good foods. The problem most people have is quantifying the reward. They eat one stick of celery and then eat twenty-five chocolate chip cookies. I reversed the process by eating only four cookies followed by eight slices of apple (one apple, cored, and sliced). By always having some fruit right after the sweets (and I mean immediately after—I slice the apple and put it on the plate with the cookies), I've learned to think of the taste of apples whenever I'm confronted by cookies. Like Pavlov's dogs salivating when they heard the dinner bell, I react to cookies by thinking of the taste of apples.

Now, there is a problem inherent in this association of tastes. You can have it work the other way around: you might think of cookies whenever you see an apple. But at least you're now considering good food right along with the bad, and the thought of your list should be enough to curtail any overeating of the sweets. I say "should be," but you've got to make that list work for you by reviewing it every night or every other night. See how much good food you can get on the list and how much bad food you can get off it.

The next step is to associate the taste of good foods with other good foods. That way you cut down on your inner urges for sweets. Fortified by your mental or physical list, you should be able to do this good-good association at least once a day. And that's one more time you eat something good, plus one more time you avoid something bad!

Cleaning your teeth

Eating something good does more than help your waistline. It also helps you protect your teeth. Naturally, you should brush your teeth after eating, but if you can't get to it right away, which foods would you think are better to have eaten last: fruit or pie, vegetables or candy, nuts or ice cream? Obviously, it makes no sense to have the sweets last. The sugar remains on and between your teeth. Perhaps by eating an apple afterward you'll at least avoid that cavity-producing act.

Cleansing your mouth

Remember how your mouth feels about fifteen minutes after eating ice cream or drinking milk? Not too pleasant. But fifteen minutes after eating an apple, your mouth doesn't taste too bad. Yes, it's still better to have brushed, but every little step helps. Eating good foods last helps rinse and cleanse your palate and mouth.

Check your list to find those foods that make you feel like a platoon of soldiers has been marching through your mouth. Avoid them as meal-enders or snack-enders.

More why . . .

Are you using food as a reward for accomplishing some task? If so, you could be in trouble, because there are always so many things that must be done for which a reward might be given: taking out the trash, doing the laundry, cleaning the house, and so forth. Not to mention all those things you must do at work.

You might say, as one young woman did, that you're only using food as a reward for one special task. Fine. I'm only pointing out that this behavior pattern is very easy to extend and expand into other areas. Pretty soon, you find yourself seeking out a sweet reward just for getting up when the alarm goes off in the morning.

Do you reward yourself because no one else does?

Does it feel like you're being ignored at work? Or just not fully appreciated? Are you trying to compensate for this "neglect" by patting yourself on the back with a sweet treat?

Perhaps you're eating too much of the wrong food out of frustration with your job. This affects all of us to a certain degree. It's one reason for the crowd around the water cooler or coffee maker at the office.

Think about your list. Not just for the good/bad foods on it, but in relation to the time spent eating. Could you remove one thing you eat at work (or perhaps just eat it later on)?

Try this: stop getting that extra cup of coffee after your first one; don't go down to the lunchroom for a doughnut in the middle of the morning; restrain yourself from running to the snack shop at 3:45 each afternoon. Instead, make yourself do one more thing at your desk. Make just one more phone call. Write just one more draft of a document.

You'll find that two things happen. One, you'll begin to have a little more zip and pep because you're cutting out a few extra, unneeded calories. And two, you'll begin to work toward more recognition in your office. After all, you'll be increasing your output without one minute of overtime. The frustration you feel at work may start to disappear, and the reward of recognition by your boss may begin. (If it does not, you may be in the wrong job—in which case you should remain on your new diet plan to help you in your search for a new position. It's a sad fact that employers are more likely to hire thinner people for almost every job. No matter how one might try to legislate non-discrimination, you cannot help but consider that a heavy person isn't going to act in as energetic a manner as a light person. I'm not saying this is true—by the way, it isn't—I'm simply pointing out that the misperception is built into society's view of overweight people.)

The holiday fill-up

Something else that may make your list longer than you want it to be is an act that was repeated at regular intervals when you were growing up. The holiday feast. All the relatives gather together and cook up enough food to serve the armies of several emerging nations. Plates are loaded with heaping helpings of food, and some of the cooks watch to see if you sample an item that they made.

"Aren't you having seconds?" asks cousin Martha. "You'll have some more, certainly," says Aunt Jane. And so forth. Some of the males brag about the number of helpings they're having, as if in competition.

Somehow it gets into your mind that overeating is good. Or good manners. Or good for you in some way. That "stuffed" feeling becomes associated with good times, good friends, and good food.

When you're growing up, you can get stuffed with food and it can be a pleasant experience. You can even burn off the excess calories and have your stomach readapt to the smaller amounts of food you normally eat. As you get older, however, your body tends to hold onto those extra calories. And you become more accustomed to filling your stomach to that stuffed point.

Look at your list and see if those childhood experiences are reflected in the food you eat these days. If you find, as I did, that your current eating habits are in some way an attempt to bring back that nice, safe, secure feeling you once enjoyed at the holiday dinner table, you are one step closer to being free of the past. Now that you know what you're seeking, you can take more care to build up your current relationships so as to provide those good feelings without involving overeating.

"Do like Mommy and Daddy . . ."

Are you eating just like your parents? If they taught you to eat slowly and eat properly, you're overweight for some other reason. But if they simply performed their own poor eating patterns in front of you, you might now be paying a price for it.

When you were small, you were urged to grow big and strong, and you wanted to grow bigger to make your parents happy. So you ate. You also wanted to grow strong to compete with your schoolmates, some of whom were always winning because they were bigger, stronger, faster, or tougher than you. So you ate.

You were taught that bigger and stronger kids could "win" arguments simply because they were bigger. You learned that, on the playground at least, might makes right. Even if the teacher was looking and punished the offender, it was still the bigger, stronger person—the teacher—who "won" the dispute.

You wanted to be the one who was in charge, the one in control. You might even have turned on someone smaller than yourself, in emulation of the bigger kids. If you were given the right role models at home, you didn't continue this practice.

But what you might have done is continue emulating the way your parents behaved toward food. They exerted a tremendous influence on you in numerous other ways: the way you speak, the way you think . . . even your taste in music and books could reflect your parents' attitudes (you may have chosen to rebel and take to activities they disliked, but they still influenced you even in this decision, if only in reverse).

There is even the possibility that you are currently eating too much and too often in an attempt to somehow grow bigger than your parents. You had times when you felt like that when you were growing up, so why not now? Sure, it's unrealistic, but so are lots of things people do and believe. Look at your list and see if any thoughts on this matter come into your mind.

Even if being able to dominate your parents isn't one of your motives in overeating, you may still be trying to please your parents, to gain their respect and admiration. You used to do this by eating, so you may unconsciously be trying to continue doing it. It may sound illogical, but it can often be true. Look at your list again. Can you see if this might be true in your case?

There is nothing wrong in either of these cases. You are perfectly normal if this is happening to you. To a certain extent, this happens to everyone. The only thing we're concerned about is how it might affect your weight, and that's the only reason we're delving into the past like this. (If you were suffering from some mental disorder because of your past, you'd have other problems besides being just a few pounds heavier than you are now. And you probably would have stopped reading by now anyway—this kind of discussion would very likely be too uncomfortable.)

What about your friends?

Examine your list with this in mind: are you eating as you do because you're trying to be like someone you admire? Sometimes it happens that we meet an extraordinary individual who seems to embody all that we wish for ourselves. This infatuation usually doesn't last, but it can be powerful while it is taking place.

You may find yourself using phrases or words that this other person uses. Certain ways of speaking are adopted. The same is true for some gestures.

But if none of this is possible, you might start trying to eat like this other, "ideal" person. Even if this person eats a relatively safe and sane diet, you may be adding pounds because you're mixing your diet with someone else's.

Watch your list and see if there are strange new foods appearing there for "no reason." It often helps to compare lists over a period of time, although it is by no means necessary to do so. If you're in the least worried about whether or not this part of The Ego Diet will work for you, then keep your lists and review them once a month.

The Thorstein Veblen complex . . . (who?)

This might also be called the show-off syndrome. It revolves around a book written in 1899 by the American economist, cynic (some would say realist), and sociologist, Thorstein Veblen. In his landmark work, *The Theory of the Leisure Class,* Veblen laid bare all his frustration and anger toward those who have money but who don't do anything useful with it. Among other things, Veblen had this to say:

> The walking-stick serves the purpose of an advertisement that the bearer's hands are employed otherwise than in useful effort, and it therefore has utility as an evidence of leisure.

He also added a phrase to our language with this observation:

> Conspicuous consumption of valuable goods is a means of reputability to the gentleman of leisure.

Now, what does this have to do with your list of foods and The Ego Diet? Well, it just might be that you are eating to show off your ability to afford so much. Or to display your familiarity with many rich delicacies. Or to make others envious of your being able to dine out in expensive French restaurants.

Take a peek at your list and see if you have to admit to eating as a form of seeking status. Do you go out to eat at places with very rich food so you can brag about it the next day? Did you learn about wine in order to appreciate it, or to show off your knowledge while conspicuously consuming some of it?

This behavior may be curtailed by thinking of the list in relation to the face of someone you respect as it smirks at you for being so silly as to try to eat your way to respect. Or you might try something that your parents probably used to try to get you to clean off your plate. They'd tell you not to waste good food because people are starving in China (or wherever). That's too abstract a concept. But think about what those starving people would say if they saw you pigging out in a vainglorious attempt to display your worth to the world.

If I don't eat something now . . .

People have asked me about the craving they get for food when dieting. "If I don't eat something now, I'll die!" said one young woman.

I asked her if she really meant that.

"Well," she said, "yes, in a way. I mean, you do need a certain amount of calories every day, don't you?"

Certainly it is good to have your intake of calories match your needs, but hunger pangs and craving for foods are mostly in the mind. People have existed for days on water alone. It's not pleasant to cut back on food, but it isn't going to hurt you if you exercise a little common sense.

You only think you need to eat something. When you go through the refrigerator at eleven o'clock at night, you're rationalizing that you "need extra vitamins because it was a rough day." Or you say to yourself, "I deserve to have a little to eat because tomorrow I've got to get up so early to make it in for a special meeting."

Unless you've skipped a meal, in which case your body might need some fuel food, you're only convincing yourself that you're hungry because you want to taste some food. Stop. Take out your list. Study it. What could you have skipped today? What could you have substituted? Do you really need to add another item to the list right now? Why not wait until tomorrow morning, when you'll be starting a new list?

You're not a child anymore. You can now give up your childish ways of dealing with food. Take control of your life and you'll eat better. Eat better and you'll gain more control of your life.

Examine your past eating habits. Think back on the eating patterns of your parents and relatives. Do they bring back good or bad feelings? Why? Are their eating patterns harming you now? Why? Call them up and thrash it out with them over the phone. (Not at eleven in the evening, please!)

Once you trace how your eating habits began, you'll be able to control them. You won't have to respond to some inner clock that commands "Eat!" You won't have to give in when you think you're too hungry to go on.

One last tip

When you review your list, cross out the bad foods, leaving just the healthy stuff. That apple you had at lunch. The orange juice at breakfast. The toast (without jam this time!). The soup. The salad.

Concentrate on these good, healthy foods, plus the others on your list. Imagine your list comprised of only good foods. Do you think you could do it for a whole day—just eat foods that are good for you? Of course you can. You have but to try.

7

Forks Down!

THE more often you eat, the more you'll lose weight. Now wait just a minute—is that right?

Oddly enough, it is true. Naturally, the amount of food you eat is the major factor in weight loss (or gain). But all things being equal, if you eat four small meals, you'll be better off than if you eat two large meals (and you'll even be a bit better off than if you eat three normal-sized meals).

An example

Let's say you eat the same number of calories on two successive days. On the first day, you eat a Danish pastry and coffee for breakfast, but have a large lunch and larger dinner. Breakfast was 250 calories, lunch 1,100 calories, and dinner 1,400 calories.

On the second day, you have the same 250 calories for breakfast, but you have a small, early lunch, a big snack in the middle of the afternoon, and a small dinner after you get home and changed into relaxed clothes. In addition to the breakfast, you consumed 800 calories at the early lunch, 850 calories at the midafternoon snack, and 850 calories at your small dinner.

Both days have a total of 2,750 calories. Now, without making any comment on whether your body needs 2,750 calories, it is safe to say you will either lose weight, maintain your weight, or not gain weight as fast if you follow the second day's plan. Spreading out your meals can help you with your diet and you don't have to change any of the food you eat.

Why? Because you burn away calories when you digest your food, and with the many meals method you make your body digest food four times a day instead of three. Same amount of food, but your digestive system doesn't know that. So it goes to work, breaking down the nutrients in the food, sending what's good to certain parts of your body, sending what's bad to other parts.

Have you ever wondered why you weren't losing weight even though you cut out a meal? It was probably because you added some food to your remaining meals, making up the calories you cut out of the skipped meal.

As a young woman who used to be a binge dieter once said, the real question is "Do you want to continue to battle overweight or do you want to learn how to eat?"

Learning how to eat

Put your forks (and spoons and knives and hands and chopsticks) down. It's almost as simple as that.

By this I mean two things. First, you should stop each meal before you get filled up. Just put your fork down and stop eating. It's better to eat again a little later.

Second, while you're eating, put your fork down between bites. Finish each bite before you pick up your fork again. This will help you eat less. You will actually feel full after eating much less food than you normally eat. When you eat fast, the body's signals about overconsumption reach your mind *after* you've already eaten too much. The faster you eat, the easier it is to gain weight. The slower you eat, the easier it is to lose weight.

There are other benefits to putting down your fork between bites. The flavors of the foods you eat will become more pronounced. Everything tastes better when you slow down. You'll become more adept at determining what flavorings, herbs, and spices people use in their food. (This will make you a more valued dinner guest, thus saving you some money!)

Taking care to finish each morsel of food has one other potentially lifesaving feature. You are more likely to avoid choking on a piece of bone, because you are taking more care in chewing your food.

Live longer

There is some evidence to support the theory that eating slowly, almost methodically, leads to a longer life. Not all the facts are in, but some impressive statistics exist.

In one family alone, the father and son—both slow eaters—attributed their longevity in part to their eating habits. The son is 71. The father, who only just recently passed away, was 97. Lest you wonder what sort of life the father was enjoying in his nineties, I should point out that he lived in a house that he built himself, tended a fair-sized garden, and enjoyed beating his granddaughter at bowling several times a week.

Other people to whom I have spoken about this phenomenon have been surprised to think about the pace of meals, but many have admitted that their longer-lived relatives did seem to "take their own sweet time at the dinner table," as one woman put it. Another older man complained that his grandfather, who was still alive and spry, "seems to dawdle over his food." We should all have people complaining about us this way.

It's actually chic

While it may not be part of the proletarian meal ritual, eating in a leisurely manner is quite fashionable. Usually, following fashion results in some sort of pain, whether it be because of tight clothes, narrow shoes, sky-high shoes, or whatever. In this case, the long, languorous way of dining is the height of chic.

A middle-aged executive named Ralph had several conversations with me bout The Ego Diet. He complained of feeling behind in his work all the time, not so much because of the pace of his job as because of the extra weight he was carrying around. He was a bit on the paunchy side of things, and this bloated condition was affecting the way he worked.

I mentioned several facets of The Ego Diet to him, but very little seemed to help. We couldn't figure out what his problem was until one day when we went out for a bite to eat together. I've never seen anyone eat quite so fast in all my life. You've heard the expression, "he practically inhaled his sandwich"? Well, Ralph was inhaling food as he walked through the restaurant door.

After pointing out that the speed of his eating probably was a strong contributing factor to his extra weight, Ralph and I talked quietly about his attitude toward food. It seems he was always a little afraid that someone was going to snatch his food away from him. He said he somehow didn't feel worthy of having it so he gobbled it as quickly as possible. He also admitted that this feeling also encouraged him to order more food than he might normally need and to consume it quite quickly, as well.

The reasons for his feelings need not be discussed here except to say that they stemmed from his childhood experiences in which he was made to feel inferior by his father. So, in trying to live up to his father's perfectionist views, Ralph was eating to grow up "big and strong" like his father, as well as feeling guilty for not fulfilling the goals his father had set for him.

I suggested he prove to himself that his will was stronger than his father's by deliberately setting his fork down in between bites of food. This may or may not have been the advice that led Ralph to eat in the forks-down manner, but he did practice this method of eating over the next several months. His weight did go down and he did report feeling more alive and alert on the job. This, in turn, led him to feel more confident in himself, and thus more worthy. And that led him to enjoy his meals, especially at his new, relaxed pace.

He told me that he was involved in an ongoing business presentation that also entailed a lot of social functions, many of them formal. One evening, Ralph was invited to the client's home for an elegant dinner party. He did not look forward to the affair because nearly everyone at his job had gone to such get-togethers in the past without any kind of breakthrough in the business negotiations. The client—or, in this case, potential client—always asked for lots of information from the men who attended these affairs. The feeling was that he was picking their brains without giving them his business.

Ralph related how the evening turned out to be a total success for him because the next day the client called Ralph's boss and presented them with the business on the condition that Ralph be one of the primary men assigned to the job.

I wanted to know what happened and I pressed him for details.

"Well," Ralph told me, "it all seemed very straightforward. I arrived, was introduced around, and we all made idle conversation through drinks. Then we went to this huge, polished-wood dining hall and were served a seven-course dinner. I was next to my host. He kept asking me questions about this, that, and the other. Since I wasn't eating as much as before, I concentrated at first on eating even slower than usual. Then, I found it was real easy to not worry about overeating, because the guy really wanted to talk, not eat. I practically ignored my food. I even worried about offending these people because I kept leaving so much still on my plate.

"Every time he asked me a question, I either told him what I thought and then asked him for his opinion, or I just said I didn't know—and asked him for his opinion. And that was it."

"Yes, but, but," I stammered, "what happened? I mean, why did you get the business?"

"Oh, that's simple," he said with a smile. "He told me later he was waiting for someone who paid attention to him rather than to the meal."

It seems so artificial!

Putting down your fork may not appear to be a true diet method, despite the case of Ralph and his weight loss. "It seems so artificial!" said one woman I met. It may be very artificial, but it works. And if it works, then it's a legitimate means of controlling your diet. It is not what is sometimes called "a big idea." But your most successful means of diet control are those that are designed to take care of you for the rest of your life and are therefore big enough ideas as far as I'm concerned. Besides, if you add up enough small but good ideas, they are frequently more effective than one so-called big idea.

Next time you're eating, take smaller amounts of food on your fork or spoon. Take smaller sips of all beverages. You are then able to extend your moments of eating pleasure. By prolonging your appreciation of foods, flavors, and the act of eating itself, you'll be able to order less. And because you're giving your body a chance to digest your food while you're still eating, your body will "signal you" that you're full sooner.

Since your blood sugar level is being raised only by the food that's already digested, you can't feel satisfied until the food you've eaten gets absorbed by your system. Eating slowly allows this to happen while you're still at the dinner table, and you are then satisfied by less food.

Some tricks

It is harder than you might think to put down your eating tools between bites of food. Anyone can do it for a while right at the start of a meal. Without noticing it, however, you can gradually speed up your pace until you find yourself gobbling as you did before you read about the forks-down method.

There are some things you can do to make it easier to tune in on your pace of eating:

- ► Make dining more of an event by making it more formal than you're used to; eating should be an *experience*, not just a humdrum part of your everyday routine.
- ► Spend a little money on the setting and the surroundings; if going out to a restaurant (not one with overly rich foods!) helps you keep your fork down, then by all means go.
- ► Avoid eating while distracted; if something interrupts, give that your attention instead of the food.
- ► Eat while sitting down, not while standing up in the kitchen.
- ► Don't talk on the phone, watch TV, read, or eat on the run

(exception: writing letters, because it involves your hands, may help you put down your fork).

► Use your best place setting, with complete sets of utensils and a place mat; you might also try putting a flower and vase on the table with your plate.

► Take care to arrange your portions of food as nicely as possible on your plate; the pleasant presentation of food will make you feel more elegant, which will help slow you down.

► Avoid highly seasoned foods that make you move fast in order to pour water down your throat after every few bites—this hurried atmosphere will influence your pace of consumption.

A calming influence

A meal that's well prepared, attractively presented, and elegantly arranged will increase your satisfaction with the act of eating. You will savor each morsel instead of gulping it down. You will admire each portion of food instead of tearing into a heap of food.

It is actually a soothing, calming act to dine leisurely. This calming influence may be felt in some homes or restaurants where the chef and/or owners are not aiming to get your meal over with in as short a time as possible. It doesn't occur very often, but when it does, you can feel the difference during and after your dining experience.

Psychologically, it's the best thing for you and your diet . . . search out and frequent any restaurant that caters to your pace. I've found that many sushi bars are delightful in this regard. You order a small portion of food, watch a master craftsman prepare it beautifully right in front of you, and then you eat that small portion and sip some tea before ordering your next few bites. Of course, you have to like sushi to partake of this pleasant experience, but I can heartily recommend trying it without worrying too much about what it is. Don't be put off by the wrinkled noses of your less sophisticated friends.

The reason we in Western society have a bad attitude toward fresh fish is simply the fact that most of our fish isn't fresh. Sushi probably doesn't exist inland because you cannot use frozen fish and have the same delicate flavors and tastes. (I am not familiar with inland areas that may have a source of fresh fresh-water fish. In theory, sushi may be made with any fresh fish, so perhaps sushi will be enjoyed soon by people in the Midwest, too.)

Another problem with our attitude toward raw fish is the way we prepare and cook fish. Since we soak fish in gobs of batter, butter, and grease, it's no wonder that we tend to think of fish in a bad light. It's also no wonder that we consider the very thought of uncooked fish to be repulsive—if you're used to tasting the fried, greasy platters of old fish we call seafood, your taste buds are spoiled for the subtle sensations of sushi. Then, too, those of us who only eat fish that has been soaked in oil or the like, aren't accustomed to the taste of cooked fish if it's prepared without the fatty additives.

Prior to my writing *The Ego Diet,* I had a long, slowly building problem with digestion of food. For several years, I had trouble going to sleep because of stomach pains. Sometimes it was accompanied by nausea, sometimes by gas. Usually it just seemed as if a lead bar was being heated by a bonfire in my belly.

If only I had had the foresight to purchase stock in the companies that manufactured products for indigestion. My own trips to the drugstore alone would have accounted for some end-of-the-year stock dividends.

After a time, even the tablets, capsules, and syrups didn't help enough to permit me to get to sleep at a reasonable hour. I was sitting up in bed or wandering around the house in my bathrobe, sipping carbonated water in a futile attempt to quell the pain.

Finally, my wife made me see a doctor about the problem. The physician I saw was an endocrinologist, a specialist in the ductless glands of the body and the secretions they produce. He listened to my story and then showed me a couple of things about myself that I didn't know.

First, he drew a diagram of the digestive system, and traced the path of food through it. He pointed out that, as we eat, we take in air with our food. The more air, the more bloated and—sometimes—more upset we can feel. In my case, he believed I was simply more susceptible to the problem of too much air in my stomach. One way to take in less air while eating is to eat slower. I promised to do that (and it alone caused me to lose some weight, quite apart from easing a bit of the pain).

Next, he explained how some foods, like beef (the "real male American's dinner"), were very hard to digest, especially if eaten in an overcooked condition (i.e., well-done). He suggested avoiding beef, particularly at night, and to avoid having it any way except rare or medium-rare on those occasions when I just had to have it. I said that I was beginning to equate beef with stomach pain anyway, and that I'd just as soon never see another steak again. (I've since been able to eat meat without any problems, but I now order it rare or medium-rare and I still try to have it early in the day or take only a half portion if it's nighttime.)

At that time, I had been experimenting with skipping dinner. This was letting me get to sleep on time and the pain was subsiding—but only when I went for a couple of nights in a row without an evening meal. This worried my wife and my mother, both of whom thought I might make myself ill by skipping dinner.

"On the contrary," said the doctor, "it's best not to have your large meal in the evening. The European manner of having a large luncheon makes much more sense from the standpoint of proper digestion. If you find you feel better by not eating much at night, I suggest you continue not eating much at night."

So, armed with this information, I went on a plan that called for a larger lunch (which was fun for me because it seemed like I was playing hookey from work in the middle of each day) and something soothing in the evening. Now, I must confess that the "something soothing" often turned out to be a beer followed by a bowl of ice milk—but at least I ate them slowly.

I straightened out my eating patterns when I put together The Ego Diet, but I still avoided dinner. I went without dinner for nearly two years. This was frequently quite hard—not because of hunger. My body quickly adjusted to taking in all the fuel food necessary at breakfast and lunch. But social convention calls for supper, and my friends were no help at all with regard to my diet. I found that saying I was doing it "on doctor's orders," in a serious tone of voice, would quell most people—after I'd explained my stomach-pain problem.

"An ulcer?" they'd ask.

At first I tried telling them the truth, that it wasn't an ulcer, but I soon discovered that the only acceptable excuse in this country for not eating dinner is an ulcer. So I lied.

"The start of an ulcer," I'd say weakly. And they would coo sympathetically and then turn back to their menus, plates, hors d'oeuvres, and so forth. I remember spending an entire meal with a friend at a Mexican restaurant during which time I had only a glass of water.

But at least I could get to sleep at night. And my stomach no longer carried around that molten-hot lead bar. Not eating at night seemed a small price to pay.

So I spent over six hundred evenings without eating, until one day I was introduced to sushi. It was actually a lunch meeting with my boss.

He had recently become a sushi freak and he insisted on taking me to his favorite place, assuring me that I could have a "regular lunch" with just a sample of sushi on the side.

I ordered something tame like teriyaki chicken, which was fine, but on the side he ordered a meal's worth of sushi. I figured I had nothing to lose but my appetite, so I tentatively bit into something called a cucumber roll. It was delicious! I didn't care what was in it, I just wanted to eat more of it. The "rolls" at sushi places usually feature crab meat plus rice, with cucumber, avocado, and other fresh goodies. I found you can also have tuna roll, California roll, the "house" roll (differs with each sushi chef), and some exotic versions I've not yet tried. The sushi itself, with a beautiful slice of very fresh fish on rice, can be dipped into various sauces, none of which, it soon developed, upset my system.

The way I found this out was by wanting some sushi so badly one night I just said the heck with it and went ahead and ordered some. "I'll regret this," I confided to my wife, "but it sure tastes good now."

Later in the evening, as I was happily reading a book in the den, my wife appeared at the door with a worried look on her face.

"How's your stomach?" she asked.

I looked up, surprised to even hear the question.

"Fine," I said, and very nearly asked her why she was asking. Then it hit me. My stomach was fine! I ate a meal after seven in the evening and my stomach wasn't even rumbling, much less causing me any pain.

It was like being cured of a long illness. Now, whenever we can afford to do it, we go out for sushi. People tell me they always feel refreshed after having it, that they seem to think better and sharper, that it is more than refreshing on the palate and tongue, it is also refreshing to the mind. Maybe I'm prejudiced, but I must say that I agree with them. (If I could figure out how to do it, I'd write "The Sushi Diet"!)

One more reason to put down your fork

In an experiment conducted with two groups of people, some overweight men and women were joined by people who were very happy with their weight. The overweight men and women were divided evenly between the two groups, and then, in separate rooms, both groups were given a test to determine their areas of interest, what they enjoyed doing in life, what hobbies they had, and so forth. In other words, the test was easy and fun to do. Both groups were kept busy for about an hour.

At the end of the test, one group was told it was a half hour earlier than real time. The other group was told it was a half hour *later* than real time. Both groups were then offered some cheese, crackers, and other snacks.

The eating pattern of the people who were happy with their weight was not unusual. They simply ate whatever amount pleased them without gorging themselves.

The overweight people in the group that had been told it was earlier than real time also displayed no unusual eating pattern, although some of them tended to keep on nibbling until nearly everyone had left.

But the overweight people who thought it was a half hour *later* than real time ate nearly twice as much as anyone else. They consumed more of the food and ate at a faster rate.

Why did this happen? When the overweight people in the second group—the group which was convinced it was a half hour later in the day than it really was—heard the time, they thought it was closer to dinnertime. The overweight people in this group were reacting to the fact that the clock "said it was time to eat."

Don't be ruled by the clock. Put your fork down before you even start eating. Ask yourself if you're truly hungry, or if you're eating because the clock shows it's near mealtime.

By putting down your fork, you'll be learning to respond to your physiological needs. If you react to outside stimuli, you will gain weight. If you use your ego, you'll learn to master all external influences —and you'll lose weight.

8

The Slower The Better

"I'VE found a new diet and I've already lost seventeen pounds in two weeks!"

"It's only been five days since I started this diet and I've lost eight pounds!"

"I lost thirty pounds in a month!"

"I lost another three pounds . . . !"

How many times have you heard stories like those? Lots of times, I'll bet. Perhaps you've even had occasion to say things like that yourself.

Bragging about rapid weight loss is one of America's favorite indoor sports. There's only one problem with rapid weight-loss programs that sound too good to be true. They *are* too good to be true. Or at least they're too good to be true for long.

What happens to most people who lose a lot of weight in a short period of time? They gain it back. And when they do, you somehow don't hear about it. The bragging stops. And the gossip starts: "Did you see Mary? She's gained back a *lot* of weight!"

This whole situation is analogous to the bragging some people do over winning in Las Vegas. You always hear about it when they win. You almost never hear about it when they lose. Yet Las Vegas seems to be going strong and making a profit despite all those winners.

The "diet-talkers"

The people who tell you about their weight loss, but forget to mention any gain, I call diet-talkers. Alice was one of these. She periodically went on a serious crash-diet program, even to the point of paying clinics for weight-loss counseling and diet plans. She would dutifully follow the meal and exercise program and report for the supervised weigh-ins. And we, her friends, would then hear about the result:

"I lost another three pounds!" she'd tell us one week. "I'm down four more pounds!" she'd say to us the next.

Oh, the weight did come off, no mistake about that. It's just that when the crash diet was through crashing she went back to her regular eating habits. And, of course, she gained weight right up to the point at which she felt it was time to go on another crash diet program. Soon we would begin hearing the all-too-familiar refrain, "I lost another three and a half pounds!"

If you added up all the pounds Alice lost in one year, you would have a number that was higher than her total weight.

Her problem was one that a great many people share. The search for speedy weight loss accounts for the constant invention of new diet plans, because the person seeking fast weight loss isn't likely to remain on the diet. After gaining back the weight lost, he or she blames the previous diet plan and immediately hunts down a new one.

Alice wanted all her excess weight to be gone in a few weeks. If she had been able to follow The Ego Diet, she might never have needed to go on another unhealthy crash diet. It may be that many people are not aware of the dangers they face by putting their bodies through the rigors of the reduce-gain-reduce cycle. If they *are* aware, then they are foolish to be taking such chances (read the section in Chapter 2 about fatty deposits building up in your arteries).

Perhaps impatience is something we as a society are building into our souls these days. We seem to instill a feeling in our children that whatever one wants is available. There was a time when the pace of life was slower, a time when some of today's modern conveniences were not available. Don't get me wrong; I'm a child of the modern age, too. And I, too, have rushed into lots of things. But when it comes to my body, one of the things I rush into is the library, to look up what other people have done in the past. While I may not follow all the expert advice I find there, at least I am aware of that advice.

Pay attention to this warning: Do not go on a crash diet except under a doctor's care and guidance. Whether you take my word for it or look it up to confirm it, crash diets are dangerous.

Slow down

Anybody can follow a rigid diet plan and lose weight fast in the first week or two. But can you stay on a rigid diet plan (even one with a built-in calorie curve to compensate for a gradual shift to weight maintenance) for fifty weeks? A hundred weeks? Two hundred?

Bet you can't do it.

That's a pretty safe bet because most peole don't remain on any diet plan that involves a crash weight-loss regimen at the start.

However, you *can* stay on a slow weight-loss diet plan. If you start by cutting back only 100 calories (about seven teaspoons of sugar—the amount you might be using each day in your cups of coffee), you're on your way to steady weight loss. Slow, sure. But steady.

A day at a time

The prospect of remaining on a diet plan for the next ten years is horribly frightening to some people. For myself, I like the idea of being on my diet plan for the rest of my life, but that has a lot to do with the fact that I now do not have pain accompanying me everywhere I go, and my diet is partly responsible for the cure.

You might be among those who are terrified of a decade or more of dieting. Don't be afraid. You only have to go on The Ego Diet for today.

That's right: today. Make certain you stay on your proper eating schedule one day—365 times a year. Wait! That's not a trick. Think about it. You can go another twenty minutes without eating, can't you? Fine. Do it. Meanwhile, drink a glass of fruit juice. It'll be digested inside of twenty minutes. Then, even if you eat an unhealthy meal, you won't be quite as hungry, because of the juice; so you'll eat less. Next mealtime, wait twenty minutes again.

Don't contemplate the future of your diet plan. It doesn't matter what you think is going to happen tomorrow. You can't lose weight tomorrow, just as you can't lose weight in the past. The only time you can lose weight is right now. Just remain faithful to your ego's urgings and refrain from having that extra helping, that dessert, that snack. Just for today.

Then, get up the next morning, stretch, make breakfast, and repeat your diet plan for just that day.

Just some kind of a stunt

A man pointed a finger at me when I was speaking about The Ego Diet and said, "That's just some kind of a stunt. Nobody can lose weight every day for the rest of his life."

Absolutely true. But a diet doesn't necessarily mean losing weight. The Ego Diet is just as concerned with your ability to maintain your weight. Sometimes not gaining pounds is a bigger victory than weight loss.

The Ego Diet is not a stunt, although I'm not above resorting to stunts that lead to healthier eating habits and healthier people. And losing a tiny bit of weight each day for a year is so much easier, so much healthier, and so much more likely to be permanent weight loss that, stunt or no stunt, I'm happy to recommend this process to everybody.

Oral gratification

Every baby goes through what is called the oral stage (usually the first year to eighteen months of life), during which time the primary consideration in life is feeding. This stage is an extremely important period in the development of every individual. So important, in fact, that many researchers believe certain personality traits that are evident in adulthood had their beginnings during the oral stage. It is during this period that babies learn to associate satisfaction with feeding (and the sucking that goes with it—this accounts for the prevalence of thumb sucking at later stages of childhood; it is an attempt to feel as safe, loved, warm, and protected as one did during the oral stage).

This association of eating with feeling satisfied, protected, and contented is something that stays with us all our lives. It does so to a greater or lesser degree depending on the individual, but it is always present to a certain extent.

Many people develop a need for oral gratification in their daily lives. This can lead some people to eat far more than they need, resulting in excess weight. Try this experiment. The next time you're hungry, take out a few pieces of gum, place the first piece in your mouth and chew. As soon as the gum loses a bit of flavor, toss it out and pop in another piece. Repeat for a whole pack. You might go through a pack of five sticks in a short time this way—anywhere from fifteen minutes to an hour, depending on whether or not you're using sugarless gum (which loses its flavor faster).

Now, two things should be evident. First, you should know if you can satisfy your need for oral gratification just by chewing something flavorful. And, second, you might be getting a feeling of "overkill" as concerns the artificial flavors in all gum. If you don't have this feeling, that's fine, because you now have a safe, sure way to keep on your more healthful diet. When you get the hunger pangs for a snack, use gum instead. If the flavor of the gum isn't really crucial to your oral satisfaction, that's great, because you may be one of the lucky ones who need only the act of chewing to become satisfied between meals.

You might be able to obtain oral gratification from chewing paraffin wax. It's cheap, it's noncaloric, and it's possible to hold a larger wad of it in your mouth without looking like a schoolyard urchin whose bubble gum is bigger than he is.

My father used to chew paraffin wax when he was a kid. Not only was it much cheaper than gum—a real consideration for a depression-era family of five—but it also had the distinction of having every bit as much flavor (none) when reused. Paraffin wax may be kept in a glass in the medicine cabinet just like false teeth. As long as it's kept clean, it may be safely reused over and over.

My dad related a lovely story to me one day after I came home from school in a bit of trouble for chewing gum in class. He said that teachers have been asking pupils to get rid of their gum in classrooms ever since there were teachers in classrooms and kids with gum. There are, however, only a few ways the teachers can enforce the rule.

"Swallow that gum, young man," is one reaction. In which case, you simply do as you're told, the wax being, if anything, less harmful than the gum.

More common, however, is the stern command to "get rid of that gum." This is how my father told me he responded when he was a schoolboy: he calmly took the wax out of his mouth, told his teacher politely that he'd save it for later, and placed the lump of wax in his shirt pocket. The teacher looked on in amazement, then finally assumed that his parents would be more upset with my dad than he, the teacher, was at that moment. Class resumed. The other kids looked puzzled. My dad just had a smug smile. He knew that all he had to do was rinse off any lint that might have gotten on the wax and his chewing piece would be as good as new.

Satisfy the urge to eat

The idea behind chewing something is simple: get your mouth moving and your taste buds tingling so you will have the sensation of eating without the intake of fattening foods. There are other ways to satisfy your oral urges. One of them has been the subject of intense debate and much legal action over the past few years: smoking.

Using tobacco

Some people take up smoking as a means of controlling their eating. A great many more find that they gain weight after giving up smoking. The fact is that smoking is a form of oral gratification that may or may not help you to stop eating so much. Even if smoking does help you cut back on your intake of food, it is such a dirty and potentially dangerous practice that no one recommends it as a diet plan unless making a frivolous or satirical suggestion (columnist Fran Leibowitz has created a "high-stress diet" that she says will help anyone lose weight; it involves getting yourself into such difficult predicaments that you will smoke seven or eight cigarettes in a half hour and thus be much too distraught to eat anything).

Smoking stains your teeth, dirties your hands and clothes, ruins your drapes and carpets, and costs too much money besides. But people still continue smoking, at least in part because addiction to tobacco is actually harder to break than addiction to heroin (I'm speaking here from the standpoint of the physical properties of the addiction, not from the severity of the withdrawal symptoms; anyone who has seen videotapes of a heroin addict going "cold turkey" knows what hell looks like).

If you don't smoke, don't start. The minor benefits you might derive from smoking's oral gratification are far outweighed by the dangers to your health.

It is sometimes important to remember that some diet methods are just not worth your time or effort. It is actually healthier to remain five or ten pounds overweight than to endanger your life with smoking or crash diets. Drastic measures are not the answer. It is so much better to lose weight slowly and naturally and just keep it off.

If gum doesn't work and you can't stand the sight of paraffin wax and you know smoking is going to hurt you, what's left? Chew on a pencil. Invest in a couple of boxes of cheap pencils and put teeth marks all over them. When they get too ratty, toss 'em.

Nibble on your key chain if you have to. If you wear glasses, take them off and slip one of the arms into your mouth. If you don't wear glasses, get some sunglasses.

Do what you have to do, but seek out your oral gratification somewhere else besides food.

Tips for slow-but-sure weight loss

Some of the tips in this chapter are obvious. Some are ingenious. All of them will work, but not all of them will work equally well for you, so you might want to try a few of them to see which methods help you the most. Even the ones that work well for you may not ever become habitual, so try another one—even one that doesn't sound like it has a chance of helping you. You might be surprised at the result.

There is something to be gained from trying almost any healthful diet tip. If it works, you've got a whole new way to help your ego reinforce your own desire to eat right and stay at your ideal weight and figure. If it doesn't work, nothing lost. All that happened was that you had to shift to one of your "fallback positions"—the diet method that always seems to work to remind you to eat right. Like waiting twenty minutes before eating. Or pinching yourself to test for fat. Or looking in the mirror. At least you have tried a new way to control your urge to eat, and the attempt itself delayed you from eating something bad even if it didn't succeed in stopping you. If it just convinces you to cut your portion in half, you'll be moving in the right direction.

Does "will power" scare you? Then forget it

I maintain that you have as much will power as the next person. You just need to exercise it. Still, the term itself bothers some people. So forget about using will power. Just stay on your healthy diet for one day. One full day, morning to sleep. That's all. Even someone with "no will power" can do that.

Next morning is something you don't have to worry about. Your will power doesn't have to stretch that far. You only have twenty-four hours to stay on your healthy diet. And eight of those twenty-four hours are spent sleeping. *Each day is a new diet that lasts only one day.*

A middle-aged lady named Wendy once contradicted me on every point I was making about The Ego Diet. The only problem was that she made the same point over and over again: she kept insisting that she had no will power at all.

"Whenever I see a pastry or some candy, I go right over and have some," she said. "I don't want to do it, but I can't help it. I just eat what I'm not supposed to eat because of something inside."

To which I said, "Hogwash!"

"Wendy," I told her, "you are a liar." Her eyes widened in astonishment. "You can control your actions just as well as I can," I said. "You just don't want to stop eating, so you made up this silly story about not having any will power. If you don't like the term 'will power,' so be it— call it something else. But whatever you want to call it, you're just lying to yourself about not having the gumption to cut your sweet-eating in half. Look, why don't you change that monologue you recite to yourself every time you feel the urge to eat a sweet." She was shocked at my tone of voice and was on the point of walking away, but my comment about her monologue made her pause.

"What do you mean?" she asked hesitantly.

"You say something like this to yourself when you see a candy store, don't you: 'I know I shouldn't eat that, but since I don't have any will power, I can't really help it; without will power, I just can't stop myself.' Isn't that about it?" I asked.

Her eyes widened again as she nodded "yes."

"Okay then," I said, "try saying this to yourself: 'I know I shouldn't eat this, but I'm a hog and so I will eat it.' Now, how does that sound?"

"That's not true!" she said loudly.

"Uh huh," I said. "How about this, then: 'I know I shouldn't eat this, but I'm such a human garbage disposal I might as well stuff it in no matter what my waist and thighs look like.' Do you like that one any better?" I was being cruel to her, but I always get annoyed with people who tell me The Ego Diet won't work for them because their will power doesn't work.

"I don't have to put up with this kind of talk," she said.

"That's true," I agreed eagerly. "But Wendy, think about how just those words are already making a difference in the way you think about sweets. Whether you call it will power or not, you have to admit that *you* are giving yourself the permission to eat the sweets; you're giving permission in the form of an excuse—by making up that line about not being able to control yourself. If *you* tell yourself you're a pig for wanting another pastry, suddenly you stop thinking about eating and you get angry. What are you mad at? The truth? Or are you mad because you just tricked yourself into not gobbling down the pastry? Either way, you just found a way to stay on a more healthy diet. And the beauty of it is that you can set your own pace and run your own controls. And damn it, Wendy, I call that will power."

Wendy has lost fifteen pounds since that time. It took her nine months to do it, but her loss, although slow, was sure. And so far, the excess weight has stayed off. Every now and then Wendy tells me she has never forgiven me for saying such nasty things to her. She also blames me because she is no longer able to think pleasant thoughts about French pastry. "Every time I see some pastry," she says, "I see this enormous pig's head looming in front of me."

"Well," I replied, "you can always switch to cookies and gain all that weight back again."

Wendy hit me on the arm. Then she took her newly trim body and hightailed it back to her newly appreciative husband.

Refuse food, even from Mom

It is tempting, especially if you're on a budget, to accept food from friends and relatives. "Here, we had some leftovers so we brought them along for you." A nice thought, but it probably won't help your weight. What tends to happen is this. You want to make use of the free food, but you don't want to waste what you've already bought. So you end up eating both. Not all in the same night, of course, but over a period of a couple of days. That free food turned out to cost you an extra pound of flab around your middle.

It may be difficult to do it, but you should try to turn down all offers of food. It doesn't matter who makes the offer: a co-worker, your boss, or even your mother.

"But I spent hours baking it just for you," is something moms are fond of saying. The old guilt trip. Still, you should turn down the offer. Refuse the "free" food.

All right, what if you just can't bring yourself to say no to some of these people? What should you do with the food? Feed it to the dog. Give it to someone else, like a bum in the street. Throw it away (especially if it's a rich dessert). Just don't keep it around to muck up your healthy diet. Yes, I was also raised to believe it's a sin to waste food. But which is the greater waste: bloating up your own body, or keeping yourself on your slow 'n' steady course (even if it means tossing a cake or casserole into the trash)? I say it's more a waste to eat unneeded food. Perhaps you can convince your relatives to donate their extra food to organizations that can give it to the needy.

I once spoke to a young man who was getting married the next day. He was so worried about his weight that he asked me what he should do about eating at the wedding reception:

"Should I eat the wedding cake?" he asked.

"No," I responded. "I never recommend eating entire cakes under any circumstances." He laughed, but I could see he was concerned. It turned out he had lost twenty-five pounds prior to proposing and he was very worried about gaining it back. "If you're really bothered about eating one slice of cake," I said, "why don't you clear this up with your fiancée first? I'm sure she'll be very understanding. After all, she wants you to be at your best weight, too. Besides, you can easily take a small bite of your cake while everybody snaps some photos of you, then put your plate down and leave it down. That won't hurt you and you'll have maintained tradition."

I found out later that both he and his bride did exactly what I suggested. By each having just one bite of cake, they both firmed up their mutual resolve to help each other stay healthier in their eating patterns.

Pat yourself on the back

Whenever you manage to slow down your eating without worrying about going on a crash diet, congratulations are due from you to yourself.

Go ahead. Tell yourself you were great out there. It wasn't easy, but you pulled it off again. If it helps reinforce your will to take it slow and steady, gush all you want.

Walter, a writer who came to see me because he had talked to David, the poet who lost weight and then maintained his perfect weight through the thinking-thin method in Chapter 4, told me he responded best to positive reinforcement.

"I enjoy staying on my diet," he told me, "because I get a chance to pat myself on the back every time I resist the temptation to eat something bad. I find it's really good for my writing to review all the good things I've done, how terrific I am, etc., just before I begin to write."

You might find you do your best work if you mentally list all the good, healthy decisions you've made in the past days or weeks. Do this just before going to work and/or just prior to tackling a particularly difficult task.

If you must use the scale

You don't need scales on The Ego Diet. You know when you're gaining or losing weight. You can feel it, see it, pinch it. Besides, your clothes don't fit. So forget the scales.

Now, for those of you who have been secretly weighing yourselves . . . you might as well know how to do it properly. The following method will make your diet easier.

If you're going to keep track of your weight, do it over a long period of time so you don't get discouraged about losing too few pounds. If you weigh yourself more than twice a month, you're overdoing it.

Give yourself a break—don't get on the scale when you're feeling fat, when you've just finished eating, when you're retaining water, or when you've got forty dollars in nickels in your pockets.

If you calculate how much weight you're losing per week, you'll get depressed. If you simply measure how much weight you've lost overall, you'll be happier. But your calculations shouldn't stop with pounds and ounces. You should also calculate how much better you feel with a few pounds off. And don't forget the fact that you're not taxing your heart as much by carrying around less weight, so you'll probably live longer.

Cleo, a career woman I met at a party, told me that she had charts of her weight pasted to her bathroom wall. She got on the scales twice a day and made a note of the result. I remarked that her method probably worked very well while she was on a crash diet, but that it was probably upsetting at other times. She looked a bit surprised, then admitted that she only used her charts when she was on a special, crash-type diet.

I talked with her about The Ego Diet and even followed up the conversation by sending her some of the rough drafts of this book. About eight months went by before I heard from Cleo again.

"I never weigh myself anymore," she told me. "You got me off the scale for good."

The funny thing was that she really was only about five pounds overweight by her own estimate. Her special "twice-a-year diet," as she called it, was quite easily adapted to The Ego Diet. She found out something that is very difficult to explain to most people: that The Ego Diet is at its absolute best when all you want to do is maintain your weight. Cleo had been able to lose those extra five pounds with no great difficulty. But she always gained them back. And she was afraid of ever gaining any more weight. Hence, her twice-yearly crash diet.

By taking everything "slow but steady" on The Ego Diet, she now maintains her weight without consulting the scales.

The tortoise and the hare

If you can stop thinking of a diet as a struggle, you'll be able to maintain a healthy diet without stress. To help remember that your progress should be slow and steady, you might think back to the story of the race between the tortoise and the hare. People who go on crash diets are like the hare, off like a shot but very erratic—and the ultimate losers (but not of pounds).

Who's counting?

I don't think counting the number of days on your diet is helpful. But there is a way to reinforce each day's success. At the end of every day in which you've been able to let your ego remind you of your diet plans, take out a sheet of paper and mark on it "Day One—You Did It!" Hang it up on your wall or put it on your dresser. Then, next morning, crumple it up and toss it in the trash as you resolve to start your "new" diet that day.

Of course you'll probably remember approximately when you began The Ego Diet, and you can tell people the correct number of months or years when they ask. However, it will be much better if you simply tell them you've been on it "one day at a time." Measuring the time you're on a diet is in itself a bit discouraging because most people still think of being on a diet as some sort of punishment. On the other hand, if you can be pleased by the fact that you've maintained your healthy diet for a long time, by all means brag about it.

That dieting can be depressing is seen in the response one young woman had to her friend's innocent question about the length of time she'd been sticking to her diet:

"One month, two weeks, three days, four hours, and ten minutes," came the reply. "But who's counting?"

You don't eat for a sore knee

When you start to waver in your resolve to keep eating good food, and none of the other methods we've discussed seems to make any difference, think of this example. If you get a twinge, say, in your knee from overexerting yourself on the weekend, you manage to get through the next few days without breaking down. You even can ignore the pain most of the time. Well, that hunger pain is no different. You can treat it the same way: find something that needs doing and go do it. You'll soon be distracted.

Think about all the stuff you live with now: you don't get along with your mother-in-law; you're not paid enough; people always drive like maniacs around you; the red lights aren't timed properly to allow you to make it through without stopping; you never learned to play billiards; you don't look like those people in the James Bond movies; and there are dead leaves all over the patio. But somehow, you've made it through life anyway. So you'll make it through the diet. Just don't force things and you'll be fine.

When in doubt, don't

This works two ways: when you're in doubt about eating something because you're not sure if it's good for you, don't eat it. You can always have it later should it turn out to be healthy rather than harmful.

On the other hand, if you're under the illusion that by holding back from eating you'll lose weight faster, then don't wait: eat something. Try to make it something good for you, or at least something neutral (like some of the trail mixes—with carob chips, raisins, sunflower seeds, and the like). Your body works better if it digests lots of little "meals" rather than a few larger ones, and if you've just eaten something good you won't be as hungry for something bad.

For a full discussion of the matter of skipping meals, see Chapter 9.

Oops!

No matter how good you are, there will come a day when you blow it and pig out. You'll feel bad about it afterward, and you might want to remember how you feel so you can prevent it from happening again, but don't get down on yourself for the slip. It happens. Just go back to a healthy diet for one more day—then one more day, and one more day . . .

You will be making a mistake if you try to make up for the extra calories by cutting out some food altogether. That's not the slow-but-steady method. Besides, your stomach will actually crave more food later on because of your pig-out session. So feed it. Just make sure you feed it good food instead of bad, and in very small quantities. Keep your digestive system going with several good things: fruit, vegetables, and grain. Avoid the kinds of foods that started the binge in the first place. Next day, add in some protein (fish, eggs, cheese, meat), and you'll be back on your healthy diet.

And cheer up. Things could be a lot worse. You could have been on one of those diet plans that calls for specific foods at each meal. With The Ego Diet, you can get back in control just like that.

9

Skip A Meal? Me?

SOME people would do just about anything to avoid missing a meal. They'd beg, borrow, or steal to get their eats. They'd lie to get out of some other activity in order to go eat. And they'd be the first to kill over food in an emergency situation.

It is possible to become fixated on food. Sometimes people see food as the solution to all problems. It isn't, but the satisfaction they derive from eating helps them overlook all kinds of other problems.

For individuals in this emotional/psychological condition, the kind of food they eat usually isn't very important to them. The way their food is prepared usually isn't very important to them. The manner in which they consume their meals is of little concern to them in most instances. And the same goes for the speed of eating.

Are you fixated on food? Ask yourself the following questions to get an idea of how you stand:

- ► Do you use a bar or nook instead of a formal dining area for most meals at home?
- ► Do you frequently skip the preparation of meals at home in favor of grabbing "a quick bite" out somewhere?
- ► At home, is your regular eating place worn or dirty in spots?
- ► Do you tend to hurry through your meals as fast as possible?
- ► When the clock says it's near your regular eating time, do you stop whatever you're doing to go eat?
- ► Do you like "all you can eat" restaurants or "buffet line" style restaurants better than regular order-from-the-menu restaurants?
- ► Do you talk about food more than other people?
- ► If other people don't finish everything on their plates, do you make an attempt to get the remaining food for yourself?
- ► Can you receite from memory the menus of the fast food places in your area?

Obviously, if you answered "yes" to a couple of these questions, you're not fixated on food. But if you answered "yes" to a great many of them, you might have an overreliance on food. You might do well to reread Chapter 6 to see if you can discover the source of your feelings about food.

Even if you are not one of the relatively few people who are fixated on food, you may still find it quite difficult to try skipping a meal. Although you may not remember it right away, you undoubtedly have missed a few meals in your life. Some personal crisis is the most common cause of having to skip a meal. If you suddenly had to take someone to the hospital, you might have missed a meal without even being aware of it. If you were involved in a minor traffic accident, the same thing could have happened.

On the other hand, it might have been good news that caused you to miss a meal. Finding out at the end of the day that you're getting that long-sought-after raise can make you so excited that the feeling of hunger doesn't have a chance to compete for attention.

Getting really wound up in a personal project can also cause you to forget about eating. Have you ever gotten involved in painting an apartment or moving furniture? It has happened to me on several occasions. Time goes by so quickly because your mind is on other things besides the clock. Time only goes slowly when you're aware of the passing of time. Someone once said that time is relative . . . a length of time is either long or short depending on whether you're sitting on a hot stove or looking at a pretty girl.

At any rate, one way or another you've probably missed a meal. When you did, you were surprised to find that you didn't get stomach cramps or hunger pains or suffer from nervous exhaustion. None of those things happened, nor would they be likely to happen even if you missed a couple of meals. For some reason, Americans think that skipping a meal is odd, twisted, disturbed, communistic, and/or will lead to grave illness. This is nonsense.

As you already know, you can live a while on water alone. Apart from that, your body may not even need three regular meals a day. Again, as you already know, eating a smaller amount of food spread out over four or five minimeals will fill you up just as much as eating a larger amount of food in three large meals.

Isn't skipping a meal unhealthy?
No. It depends on whether your body needs some fuel to keep going.

If you aren't doing anything that requires a lot of energy, you may be better off skipping a meal now and then.

Don't be fooled into assuming you need energy only for physical labor. If you intend to concentrate on an important document for work —or use your mental capacity in any of a number of other ways—you actually need more fuel food than when you're engaged in heavy physical labor.

It's only when you "turn off your mind" with television (a very passive activity) or idle conversation or sunbathing that you don't burn up much fuel. In this state, you might as well keep your body as healthy as possible and not cram it full of extra calories.

Is skipping contradictory to having many minimeals?

Yes and no. It is directly counter to the idea of having a lot of little meals spread out over the day. But you can afford to skip a meal if you've taken care to give your body some protein, some grain, a fruit, and a vegetable at some point during the day.

Still, even if these two methods were diametrically opposed to each other, I'd have no trouble recommending them to you as things to try. You might find that alternating between the two ideas is your best diet plan. You certainly wouldn't get into a rut that way.

What happens when you skip a meal?

When you were busy with something that distracted you from the desire to eat, hardly anything seemed to happen to you when you skipped a meal. When you deliberately try to skip a meal, you feel like your stomach is crying out to you for food. Why is that?

A great deal of your "hunger" is in your mind. You get signals from your body that you're hungry and your mind won't let you forget those signals. You begin fixating on the tummy growls and your taste buds begin working despite having nothing to work on. But these physical reactions stop the instant your mind switches over to another topic. If you get distracted from the hunger problem, you can be completely unaware of how you felt a moment before.

Once you do miss a meal, you'll find that you don't eat as much at the next meal—assuming your body doesn't crave fuel. Even if you skipped a meal because of some mental or physical activity, you might be able to eat only as much as if you had never missed a meal.

Contrary to popular belief, your stomach does not shrink because you miss a meal. Your stomach remains about the same size all the time. What happens is that your stomach becomes used to working on a smaller amount of food, so you feel much more full—that "stuffed feeling"—when you eat the next meal. This should help you eat less. If you can feel satiated by a smaller amount of food, you will be able to control your diet very easily.

Diet every other day?

Some people have been able to lose weight by eating a healthy diet one day, then going back to their old habits the next. This odd method does actually have some value for losing weight.

Since your stomach will react to the smaller amounts of food that are eaten on the "good diet" day, you are likely to eat less on the "bad diet" day which follows. I have even talked to some people who insist that their taste for better foods has increased on the every-other-day diet plan. I have my doubts about this. As you probably noticed, when people acquire a taste for the fatty, oily foods served in junk food parlors, it is often difficult to get them to appreciate the subtle flavors of food that is more sensibly prepared. Like one rotten apple turning the whole barrel bad, or like bad music driving good music out of the marketplace, bad foods tend to take over from better ones.

What happens is quite simple: your taste buds become numb and lazy. Foods that are fried in batter, butter, or fatty oils attack your taste buds. The taste of these foods is so overpowering that your taste buds don't have to do any of their work—the food just marches over your tongue, showing no mercy and taking no prisoners. You could be given a prize-winning soufflé and not notice its delicacy of flavors.

Remember what happens when you eat some foods right after something salty—for example, ice cream after potato chips? Or when you try eating an olive after taking a drink of milk? You have undoubtedly tried two foods in combination that just didn't do anything to help the flavor of either one. Well, that's similar to the effect on your taste buds of having bad food—it makes the good food unpalatable. Literally.

This doesn't have to happen on the diet-every-other-day plan, of course. It depends on what you eat on your off day. So if you're considering this plan because you intend to stuff everything but the kitchen sink into your gullet on the nondiet day, forget it. That's not the way The Ego Diet works.

Another drawback to the every-other-day diet plan is the natural human tendency to try to compensate for what happened the day before. Or to compensate for what is about to happen tomorrow. Either way, if you try to compensate by grossly altering your intake of food, you're going to hurt yourself.

If you try to cut back to an even stricter level of dieting because you had too much chocolate cake the day before, you may not give your body enough fuel to get you through the day.

Conversely, if you try to "stock up" for the semifasting you intend to do tomorrow, you risk bloating your belly (not to mention risking a stomachache).

Handled with caution, however, this plan can produce results that are slow but sure. I knew a girl in high school who used the plan to good advantage. I thought she was crazy at the time, but looking back on what she accomplished (weight loss of fifteen pounds over the course of a twenty-week semester and maintenance of her ideal weight thereafter), perhaps she instinctively knew what to do.

On her "eating days," she would have an egg, toast, and half a grapefruit for breakfast; a hamburger, fries, malted, and (sometimes) a small salad for lunch; and then whatever regular dinner her mother prepared for the family at night. On her "fasting days," she would have the same breakfast as on other days, but she would skip lunch and dinner. She had to arrange to be away from her house at dinnertime and to lie about having dinner with a friend, in order to keep her mother from worrying, but other than that her system seemed to work for her. She was never ill and always appeared to have plenty of energy, even on her fasting days.

Notice that she was still getting some protein (the egg), fruit, and grain (the toast) on her fasting days. This was either very smart on her part, or she was lucky that her mother insisted on her eating breakfast. Her body needed the fuel.

Also, by having a piece of fruit every day, she was putting something fresh into her body on a regular basis. As you probably know, it's not a good move to try eating four pieces of fruit at one sitting to make up for skipping fruit three days in a row. Actually, it's not a wise idea to try making up for anything you missed at prior meals—at least not in any one day. The best thing to do is just go back to your healthy good habits after you've disrupted your regular patterns. Your body will quickly adjust to receiving a small amount of fruit each day even if you've been skipping fruit for several days at a stretch.

In this regard, your body reacts similarly to your need for sleep. If you go without sleep for two days, you don't have to sleep for sixteen hours just to make up the lost eight hours of sleep. You can grab eight hours and be back in action with a fairly clear head.

The typical thing to do in this kind of situation is to sleep for twelve hours straight. But this just throws your system out of balance about as much as getting too little sleep. You may have noticed that you are groggy and a bit disoriented after sleeping too long. Just as with food, you should find out the amount of sleep that's best for you. If you're too tired to let your ego guide you in your decision making about food, you might blow your diet plans without giving yourself half a chance. Try to get your required amount of sleep every night.

Most people require between seven and nine hours of sleep in every twenty-four-hour period. I find I get along quite well on seven, while my wife needs closer to eight. My father needs more like nine hours. Instead of getting it in one long session, from which he might emerge a little dazed and befuddled, he sleeps for about seven hours at night and takes a nap in the early afternoons—a very sensible, albeit sometimes impractical, solution.

Can sleep substitute for food?

Because sleep is very often refreshing, some people have wondered if they can sleep a little longer and eat a little less. To the extent that lying in bed burns off fewer calories than walking around, you can say that less food is needed if you sleep longer. This hardly seems a sensible way to diet. And if you've ever tried to go to sleep when hungry, you know it's difficult to stop thinking about food. If this happens to you, by the way, get up and read a while. The hunger pains will soon disappear. (I know it doesn't seem possible, but try it.)

Still, I have talked to some people who say they have managed to skip meals by going to sleep. What they did is stay up later than usual, but without having any late-night snacks. They also grabbed forty winks when they would otherwise be eating lunch. (Again, there's the problem of napping being impractical for most of us.) These guys—all college students—had a variation on the sleep-for-food scheme. Again, it involved staying up later than usual for two nights in a row, then crashing into bed without supper the third night.

The reason this worked for them has to do with a certain biological factor called youth. Unless you're closer to twenty than thirty, you'll find this method of dieting debilitating.

Why all these warnings?

So far, I've done very little but warn you of the dangers and pitfalls of skipping meals. Why? Because it can be very dangerous. It is almost always better to eat something—even if it's a tiny amount—at your regular three or four eating times during the day.

Then why recommend the skip-a-meal method at all? Well, because it can work if you handle it properly. I found that I was slowly gaining weight at one point after I had discovered the success of The Ego Diet. At the time, I couldn't figure out why I was gaining, so I did the only thing that seemed to be available to me: I skipped a meal a day for three days each week. That did the trick. I lost the couple of pounds I had gained. Then I cut back my skipping to only two meals a week, and maintained my weight.

Now, looking back on this particular period of my life, the problem seems quite obvious even though I was blind to the cause at the time. Here's what had happened:

I worked with another writer on various projects until she left for a new job out of town. Her departure coincided with a slight lull in the flow of work. So, although I missed her personally because she had a quick wit and a ready smile, I did not notice her absence in the professional sense.

Slowly, over the next few weeks and months, the pace of the work picked up. And up. And up. Until I was hurrying in to the office at eight or eight fifteen in the morning and not leaving for home until seven or eight at night. While I enjoyed the responsibility, I will admit the pressure was a bit much.

My eating habits had to change. My body craved more fuel. I grabbed fast foods often. A sandwich here. A hamburger there. Doughnuts in the morning. A bag of nuts in the afternoon. To the extent that I needed the extra protein, some of these foods were helpful. But the habit of eating anything and everything at any hour was hard to break when the pace of work began slowing down.

I was gaining weight at that point. The work level was still higher than it had been before the other writer left, although it had tapered off somewhat. I still didn't have the time to think through the problem fully, so I did the only thing I could come up with: I skipped breakfast. This worked for me. I gradually lost the pounds and then maintained, according to the schedule I mentioned before.

There are better ways to handle weight loss and weight maintenance, but skipping a meal may work in a difficult time. You may be able to make a better decision about skipping a meal if you know which meal to skip.

Skipping breakfast

If you're going to skip a meal, breakfast is the easiest to skip. Your stomach has already gotten used to not having anything in it, and therefore it is at its "smallest." Then, too, if you're like me, you take a dim view of the morning—primarily because your view of things *is* dim. I'm not at my best after waking up. My tongue is thick, my eyes are half closed, my head weighs more than my body, and my legs move about as fast as two redwood trees. And that's on the good mornings.

With all that to contend with, you can see why many of us aren't in what you might call an eating mode early in the morning.

Unfortunately, breakfast is also the worst meal for you to skip. You are in need of fuel food to start your day, and a little protein in the morning can do a lot to help make your body respond at its best. Having a bit of good food at breakfast can also help clean your mind of the cobwebs. The groggy feeling goes away if you can get your digestive system working on something healthy.

As millions of morning-haters have discovered, getting a set routine that you can (literally) follow in your sleep will go a long way toward helping you get up, get dressed, get moving, get fed, and get out of the house.

As part of my routine, I grind coffee beans into a fine powder in an old-fashioned hand-crank grinder. This ritual serves to start my motor running. Then I "move it" with a few—just a few, mind you—exercises (more about this in Chapter 13). Next comes a shower.

All that, I find, is necessary to get me to the point of wanting to eat something for breakfast. But the effort is worth it because I always go off to work feeling bright-eyed and bushy-tailed. Prior to setting this routine, I went in to work cursing the day.

Despite it being the worst meal to skip, you can try skipping breakfast if you are careful to monitor yourself as to your energy output during the morning hours. I recommend you try skipping either lunch or dinner rather than breakfast, so you don't have as much to worry about.

You might try having a piece of toast instead of a full breakfast, especially if you usually drink coffee or juice in the morning. The grain won't hurt you (it's the butter and jam that have the calories) and it will help your stomach with the terrible acidity of the java or fruit juice.

One of my mother's women friends keeps a jar of wheat or soda crackers on the breakfast bar. In the morning, or when she feels like having a snack, she dips into this jar for a couple of crackers. That's much better than most snack items, and it's particularly good to offset the acid of coffee. This is a healthy way to deal with cravings between meals. It also may work as a substitute for a skipped meal.

It isn't necessary to refrain from eating entirely when skipping a meal. Having a few crackers and something to drink is an excellent way to satisfy your need to go through the motions of eating without adding a lot of calories. There is a potential problem with this, however. Some people find that the very act of eating—even if they're eating only a cracker—triggers their desire to consume a full meal. You'll have to test yourself on this. You may find that it is much wiser for you to cut out all food in order to make yourself skip a meal. If you find that you are able to nibble a couple of crackers without being faced with an uncontrollable desire for more food, you're fortunate.

Breakfast is the only meal that has an absolute termination point. Most of us must leave the house at a certain time in order to make it in to work promptly. Because of this, breakfast is also the only meal where a few bites of toast or crackers absolutely cannot lead you to more eating—if you time things right.

Skipping lunch

Depending on your work load, lunch is either very easy or very hard to skip. When the work pace is fast and furious, I can skip lunch even when I don't want to do so. But when things are slow, it's very difficult to skip lunch. There are several reasons why this is so.

First, you've got little to do, so you're apt to become bored. To fill the time, you sometimes go looking for a snack. Second, when it's slack, lots of people with whom you work will be busy organizing lunch get-togethers. You're likely to be asked to join one or more of them. Third, even if you refuse to accompany your friends to lunch, you're now sitting in a quiet, empty building with even less to do than before lunchtime. It's not long before you're heading out to the commissary or one of those "roach coaches" that line up in a parking lot or at curbside.

I don't recommend skipping lunch, either, but it is a better meal to skip than breakfast, especially considering the kind of lunch we Americans tend to favor. The European custom of having a large lunch, then taking a brief break from work to digest it, is much more conducive to good health than our custom of grabbing lunch on the run.

Not only do we eat too fast, we usually eat the wrong foods or foods prepared in the wrong way. Our lunches are rarely balanced meals. When was the last time you heard someone say, "Never mind about the time. We'll just grab a salad on the way." No, the word "salad" doesn't usually enter the conversation at that point. Instead, you hear "sandwich," "burger," "quick something," and so on. Skipping these things would be better for you.

Again, having something at lunchtime is better than denying yourself all food. The snack crackers should come in handy here, too. Or you might try having a liquid lunch. No, I don't mean five martinis. I'm talking about soup, dinner salad (lettuce is largely water), and something nonalcoholic to drink. A glass of milk, for example. Later on, when you're down to your comfortable weight, you can raise your caloric intake a bit by switching to milk shakes.

An aside on "comfortable weight"

When I say comfortable weight, I mean the weight at which you feel best. This is the weight that *you* feel is ideal. All through this book, I've used the term ideal weight. This might be a good time to point out that what is ideal for you may not be "fashion model thin." Or, as some would say, "fashion model skinny." Do not worry if you feel comfortable at a weight that is a few pounds over somebody's weight chart.

As already pointed out—but is so crucial it bears repeating—if you think that you are likely to gain back a few pounds, then lose them, then gain them again, and so on, then it's much healthier for you to just remain a few pounds above what some charts tell you is your ideal weight. You're the one who has got to live with your body. You're the one who must be proud and stand tall. If you can do that by accepting your body at your present weight, then please use The Ego Diet to maintain your weight, not lose weight. I still think The Ego Diet is the best method available for losing weight, but it's primary function is as a lifelong weight maintenance program.

Skipping dinner

This is the right meal to skip.

I know, I know, it's also the hardest to skip, and for many reasons.

Big dinners are a tradition in America, and tradition always dies hard. We all have trained ourselves to expect a large meal at suppertime, Charles Schulz, the man behind the comic strip "Peanuts," capitalized on this phenomenon with many strips about Snoopy, Charlie Brown's dog, and his fascination with suppertime. The play

You're a Good Man, Charlie Brown even has a song called "Suppertime."

Another reason is that suppertime is the only meal where the whole family can gather together. Lunch, of course, is impossible, but even breakfasts are often taken in shifts in order to accommodate the various school schedules and car pool schedules of all the family members. It seems a shame to suggest something that might break up the one chance for everybody to get together with one common interest. But then, from what I've seen of some households, all that might be broken up is some of the television viewing that goes along with dinner.

At any rate, if a meal is to be skipped with minimum health risk, dinner is the one. You don't need to build up fuel for sleeping. You don't usually do enough to truly digest all your food properly. And you tend to eat too much because of the distractions of too many conversations and/or the sound of the television.

This is the meal where the extra weight gets put on your belly, your thighs, your upper arms. You say you need to relax, so you have a drink. You say you're hungry after a hard day, so you load up your plate with all sorts of extras like bread, rolls, creamed potatoes, or coleslaw. You say you don't have time to make a full dinner, so you bring in chicken fried in tons of batter. You say you deserve a treat, so you have a dessert that is totally unnecessary for your health.

All of these food items are fairly harmless in and of themselves or if eaten once in a while in moderation. But you eat them all at once, and all the time. And you eat them quite fast, which doesn't allow your body to digest them well.

You also ignore that "signal" your body sends you when you're getting filled up. Not the "full to bursting" feeling you get at those holiday feasts. I'm talking about that feeling you get when your stomach has taken in just enough food to comfortably digest it—this usually comes about halfway through the typical American meal. Most people ignore it because they like the sensation of eating. Your stomach can handle more food, and obviously does, but it doesn't work at its best when you fill it beyond a certain point.

Yes, you could probably stand to skip dinner entirely every other day. Or, you could just pay attention to your body's signals and cut your evening meal in half. Do that and you'll already be using The Ego Diet in a way that might extend your life by several years.

10

The Ways Of Water

YOU cannot exist without water. It is as basic to life as air.

Water is in the atmosphere and in the air you breathe. Your body is approximately 66 percent water. Water is distributed throughout your body, and there are few bodily functions that are unaffected by water. The earth's surface is three-fifths water, close to the same percentage as in your body. Perhaps nature is trying to tell us something.

Being deprived of water is actually more anguishing than being deprived of food. After three days of starvation, hunger pains tend to disappear, although weakness sets in. A shorter period of time without water produces mental and physical disorders.

With water you live; without water you die. It's as simple as that.

But there's more to water than being part of the basic stuff of life. Water can also be your secret weapon in your battle to lose weight and maintain your perfect weight.

Using water for weight loss

It is important to consider water intake in any diet plan. Some diets ask you to count the number of glasses of water you drink each day. There are "water diets" as well as other weight-loss plans that require you to drink six, eight, ten, or more glasses of water or some water-based juice or other liquid in a given day. This will work, of course, but it can become a crash diet plan, and that's dangerous.

A dozen glasses of water in any one day won't hurt you (although there is such a thing as having too much water; it's called water intoxication), but there is a greater drawback than the possibility of using water in a crash diet manner. Drinking that much water every day can become real boring, real fast. And when that happens, your body rebels, causing a thirst for something else. Almost anything else. And before you know it, you're not drinking your prescribed number of glasses per day. In fact, you've probably abandoned the whole plan.

Instead of trying to drink a large number of glasses of water every day of the week, just try to drink one glass of water before every meal. That's it: just one glass, one meal. A pretty fair trade-off, wouldn't you agree?

That one glass of water will help fill you up. Because your stomach will be partially filled, you'll be more likely to eat less at each meal.

Water will also help clean and flush your body. It can help remove some of the mildly toxic substances that accumulate in your body. Think of it as flushing out some mild poisons. Getting rid of these unneeded substances will help you feel better, be more resistant to illness, and look better. Your face will look a bit softer and younger when you're using the water method.

A glass of water is especially needed if you intend to have some junk food. Give your body a chance to handle some clean, easy-to-digest, clear liquids prior to hitting it with a corn dog, doughnut, or something of that ilk.

Water as a control device

There is a psychological reason for having the glass of water before each meal. It serves to remind you that you are still on The Ego Diet, and it helps you remember that you are the one in control of your body, not the other way around. As you're sipping the cool, refreshing water, think about how you will not be ruled by your taste buds or your tummy. You can rely on the water to act as a control device for your healthy eating plans.

Water in place of snacks

You can use water in place of snacks, although I do this only as a last resort. If you're trying to speed up your weight loss by finding extra reasons for drinking water, then you're really searching for a crash diet. In that case, please look elsewhere. Even with the water method, slow and steady is the way that will help you more in the long run.

Using water to maintain your weight

Basically, the same methods apply to weight maintenance as applied to weight loss: drink a glass of water prior to every meal. The difference is that you may need to use water as a flushing mechanism when you've decided to eat something bad for your system.

You know how it goes: you'll be coasting through the day, not worrying about your weight or your eating patterns (at least this is how it will be after The Ego Diet becomes part of your everyday routine).

Suddenly, you're confronted with the tempting opportunity to eat something you have always loved—but which you know is not good for you. Perhaps someone brought glazed jelly doughnuts to work. Or you find yourself in the vicinity of a particularly noteworthy chili dog emporium. Or any one of a hundred other situations involving some rich, oily, or greasy food. (You can tell that I have sampled foods like this. I've even done it while still maintaining my weight on The Ego Diet. I am going to say some nasty things about this type of food later on in this book. Please believe me when I say I know how good this kind of stuff can taste every once in a while. That's the secret, though: just have food like that once a month or so instead of two or three times a week.)

Anyway, you have some no-good taste treat dancing before your eyes and, just as suddenly, little taste alarms begin going off in your mouth. "Feeeeeeeeed me!" they cry. And you do just that.

What to do after you succumb to temptation

Well, all right, let's admit that it happens. And let's also admit that one jelly doughnut will not kill you. Nor will one chili dog. True, neither is very good for your digestive system or your figure. And true, both contain lots of calories and waste materials your body could do without. But still, eating one won't bring on the end of the world as we know it.

The trouble is this: many of us find it harder to stop after eating one bad food than to refrain from eating the food in the first place.

So, use the glass of water before you eat and use another after you finish eating as well, In fact, have several glasses. Help your system adjust to the grease or oil by giving it something to use to break down the bad food.

Besides, by drinking several glasses of water after having that one bad food, you are combating the desire to have more of the unhealthy food.

Learn to taste water

Taste water? You bet. You can learn to appreciate the taste of fine water. You can make it a part of every meal, treating it with special care and consideration. It can become a delicacy, no less.

Water has flavor. It has become very difficult for you to tune in on the flavoring of water because your taste buds have been bombarded with much stronger taste sensations.

You can find water that tastes good, bad, and in-between. It's different in every part of the country. It's even different in each part of a city. You should be able to taste the difference when you're at another person's house.

To truly appreciate the taste of good water, try some bottled water. Seek out some restaurants that feature some of the imported waters. You can order one of the many varieties of bottled water to drink before your meal. After a meal is a good idea, too—especially in place of dessert. Some bottled waters contain salt, but unless your doctor forbids you to have even this small amount of sodium, I suggest you not worry about it and order the brand of water that tastes best to you. Some have natural or added carbonation and all are particularly good with a twist or a squeeze of lemon or lime.

Society's effect on our tastes

Although hunger and thirst are two of the most powerful motivators in all of human activity, they are just physical mechanisms. Thirst is just a warning from your body that your fluid level is getting low, like the warning light in your car that tells you you're running low on oil. The sensation of thirst is just a signal that is transmitted to your pharynx—the upper back portion of your throat.

Because thirst and hunger are physical mechanisms, they can be affected by our psychological actions. For example, people who lived through periods of time when they were deprived of food and water, such as people who were in political prisons in foreign countries or who lived through the depression, even now are affected by the experience. They are much more likely to engage in aspects of hoarding, always insisting on having the refrigerator fully stocked and the pantry shelves fully loaded. They are the ones who encourage everyone—not just their relatives—to eat up, and "clean off that plate." They are reacting to food entirely differently from the way you and I do.

The following experiment is an example that's much closer to our own experiences; it shows just how societal conventions and the need for status affect what we think.

Several bottles of the identical brand of beer were used in the test (right away, many of us are wishing we could have been part of the test—just in the hope of furthering scientific investigation, mind you). All labels and brand identifiers were removed from the bottles and replaced with price tags of varying amounts. People in the experiment were then allowed to sample each bottle. They were asked to describe the taste of each bottle. Invariably, people described the bottles with the higher price tags in more glowing terms of praise. This despite the fact that all the beer in all the bottles was the same.

So I suppose you might even be able to convince yourself that plain old city water has lovely properties of taste, bouquet, and so on.

What's in the water?

Depending on the mineral content, chemical additives, filtration systems utilized, and so forth, water everywhere will not only taste different, it will *be* different. If you're going to use water in your diet—and you should—make certain you can trust your supply. Some newspaper accounts of the testing of municipal water delivery systems have scared a great many people into buying bottled water for all internal uses.

Reports of rusty water have been common for decades, even in cities with good, clean supplies of water. Obviously, the rust has come from the household pipes rather than the city pipes in most instances, and this is something to avoid. Check your pipes at home to be sure you haven't been spouting rusty water and then drinking it.

Chemical dumping has affected the water supplies of many cities both large and small. You may not know if your area has been affected unless you pay a laboratory to test your water. Even then, the water could be reasonably pure on the day of the test and you could still wind up drinking impure water at a later date.

There have been incidents of sewage system leakage affecting groundwater (water that lies beneath the earth's surface and which supplies springs, rivers, and lakes). Again, if this is affecting your supply of water, you could be poisoning yourself, albeit slowly, and you wouldn't know it. And again, a lab test is only good for the day or days of the testing, not for all time.

The most upsetting story about city water came from my own town. Apparently, a few neighbors were complaining about the bad taste of their water, so one man had some samples tested. The report that came back showed that fly larvae had been present in the water. Next time you think about saving a few pennies by skipping bottled water, think about drinking the newly hatched vermiform (wormlike) feeding form of houseflies.

Before you dismiss this example as a fluke or a once-in-a-lifetime problem, consider this: there are thousands of potentially dangerous chemicals that pose a risk to our water supplies. Agricultural use of chemicals, both in additives to fertilizer and in spraying, is very high in many parts of the country. Not more than six miles from where I sit typing this sentence, helicopters were busy spraying Malathion last night. Malathion is an insecticide that is used to kill, among other things, the Mexican fruit fly. Rainwater that runs off the sprayed area will enter the groundwater.

In addition, groundwater may be affected by seepage from mines and septic tanks, and by runoff from landfills and feedlots. One estimate puts the number of barrels of brine (water saturated with salt) dumped into our underground water sources at 10 million per year. When you reflect on the fact that 20 percent of all water used in the United States comes from groundwater, you can see that you are likely to be affected.

As of this writing, the Los Angeles Department of Water and Power has a printed warning on the back of all their invoices stating that consumers may experience "turbidity" in their drinking water. Turbidity, they tell us, means "cloudiness." It means dirty water to me.

In 1975, the National Academy of Sciences was utilized by the Environmental Protection Agency to test the water supply of American cities. This study was in response to the Safe Drinking Water Act of 1974. The study showed several thousand organic chemicals to be present in the drinking water of eighty cities.

I think you're beginning to see why I scoff at those people who suggest that a puny little filter attachment to the faucet of your home will protect you from impurities in your water.

Drink the good stuff

Once you have made certain you can trust your supply of water (or you have laid in a personal supply of bottled water), drink up. Learn to be a connoisseur of bottled water. Talk about the various kinds you've tried. Find others who share your regard for the cleansing effects of a few glasses a day. While I do not recommend that you flaunt the facts about the impurities of city water, you can quietly discuss your feelings once you get to know someone.

A word of warning: People can be very stubborn about their belief that the water they drink is not potentially harmful to them. They do not want to be educated and they may get angry with you for trying to help them. People who respond negatively to what you have to say should be left alone concerning this subject. Find something else to talk about. But don't drink the water at their house. Or anything made with water.

What about beverages made with water?

Many canned or bottled fruit juices have water as their primary ingredient. While these are not as good for you as freshly squeezed juices, they are still quite healthy, if—and this is a big if—they do not contain sugar (other than the natural fruit sugar). If you wish to substitute fruit juice for water, go right ahead.

Coffee and tea contain no calories and are largely water, but they add chemical substances to your body. Even decaffeinated coffee and tea. You will not gain weight drinking these substances, but you will look and feel better if you avoid them as much as possible.

I was surprised to find out how many cups of coffee I was drinking each workday. Count your cups during the day and see if you aren't surprised at the total. I have now cut back to two cups of coffee a day, one at breakfast and another in the middle of the afternoon. When I feel the need to have more hot liquid to drink, I squeeze a quarter of a lemon into a mug of hot water. It sounds awful but tastes surprisingly nice: a kind of mellow drink, actually.

Diet soft drinks have even more chemicals in them than coffee or tea. No, you won't gain weight by drinking them either, but you're not really doing your system a favor with these things. Get some carbonated water and add some lemon or lime to it. Served in a glass with a straw, it's a rather continental beverage, and it will make all your fellow workers wonder what you're drinking (it will look like a gin and tonic, but you'll be working away, sober as a judge, even after having four glassfuls).

Drink water without drinking

Sound impossible? You can find water inside many foods. Eating these foods before meals acts in a fashion similar to drinking part of a glass of water. You get the same feeling of fullness and also give your stomach more to digest than plain water.

The foods that come most readily to mind are celery, radishes, cucumber, and lettuce. Because of its cleansing action, you should continue drinking water; the best thing you can do is combine the eating of these foods with the drinking of one glass of water.

Whichever way you decide to handle the problem, the water method should become a regular part of your eating habits. Have water before meals while dieting to lose weight; have water before meals and in larger quantity to flush your system after bad foods while dieting to maintain your weight.

One drawback to the water method

You've probably already guessed what the drawback is. If you've ever had a glass of water or a glass of beer on an empty stomach, you'll remember what happened about a half hour later. You needed to find a rest room.

So, if you decide to cleanse your system with several glasses of water, do not do so in a place without public rest rooms. This may seem like such basic common sense that it doesn't bear mentioning, but hold your judgment until you learn what happened to me.

I was involved in a multimedia art and dance presentation for the Century City Cultural Commission. My participation was supposed to be fairly minimal: just provide some visual projections to accompany a group of dancers who would be performing to prerecorded music played over a "mobile deejay" sound system.

There was no money involved and no rehearsal so I just piled as many film and slide projectors as would fit in my car and tootled over the Century City. After parking underneath the Century Towers, near the freight elevator, I unloaded the equipment and the film loops (sequences of movies which have the front spliced onto the end so that they run continuously), colored slides, liquid color wheels (plastic discs with colored oil inside, which, when placed in a slide projector, enable the globs of oil to appear to spin and undulate on the screen), and all sorts of other visual goodies.

There were about three dozen other groups of artists, dancers, and musicians involved in the event, and the whole conglomeration of us was spread out across the unfinished thirty-third floor of one of the Towers. As the sun began to settle into the sea—a glorious view from that high above the city—it became apparent that we were the only group with the one essential ingredient for competing for the attention of the hundred or so guests, politicians, businessmen, and off-duty artists: amplification. The deejay began cranking up the volume as darkness began to fall.

Now it became apparent that whoever planned this brouhaha had neglected to find out if the lights had been installed on the thirty-third floor. Most hadn't. Only the safety lights near the elevators were operating. Which meant that we had the other essential ingredient for capturing everyone's attention: light, from my projectors.

So the scene was total madness. All the participants and guests were scrunched into two areas: our noisy, sweaty, wildly colored alcove, and the hallway in front of the elevators. A video crew arrived and began taping everything in sight, which wasn't much under the circumstances.

Meanwhile—silly me—I soon started to feel the effects of the five glasses of water I had bolted down just prior to the start of the show. I left the projectors running and went looking for the men's room. There wasn't one. Hmmm. Well, I'd have settled for the ladies' if someone had cleared the way for me. There wasn't one of those, either. What the hell? It turned out the genius who set up this gig not only forgot that it gets dark at night but also neglected to ensure adequate health facilities would be available.

Oh well, I thought, I'll just make the trip down the elevator to the rest rooms in the lobby. Ooops, wrong again. A group of disgruntled and/or scared folks was milling around the front of the elevators while the video crew was taping an interview with the closed doors of one elevator . . . wait, this was insane. What was going on? Both elevators were jammed. One was stuck right here on our floor, which was why the video guys were apparently talking to the closed doors of the elevator—they were talking to the group of people trapped inside. The other elevator, according to someone who was on the emergency phone inside the elevator, was stalled down in the lobby.

Wonderful. My bladder was becoming insistent. I had to relieve the pressure, and right then.

Well, what would you do? I went to the emergency stairs, dragged one of the plastic-lined trash dispensers with me, and did what man has been doing ever since water was invented.

I went back to the dancers and began packing up my equipment. They were understandably disappointed that their source of light was disappearing, but I wasn't about to stick around for the next fiasco in that building.

But I did. After getting the equipment down to the lobby level (no, I didn't carry it down thirty-three floors; the security people in the building finally got the elevator working), I discovered that the only elevator that went from the lobby level down to the parking garage was also jammed. The event organizers pointed out to those of us with equipment that we could drive our cars up alongside the building to load. Which we did. But most of the others had made the mistake of taking their equipment down in two trips. So after loading their cars, they went back up into that foul building for another adventure. At which point the Century City meter maids arrived as if on cue and began placing parking tickets on all the cars not immediately vacating the vicinity.

I let this become my lesson in regard to the water method. Always check for rest rooms before drinking.

11

Why You Get Hungry

YOUR body is always striving for perfection. It tries to keep your temperature within one degree of 98.6 Fahrenheit (37 Celsius) no matter whether it's 20 below zero or 135 degrees above. The chemical properties of your blood are constantly being monitored as to the correct proportion of oxygen, salt, acidity, and so forth.

When you are low in blood sugar, a signal is sent to your hypothalamus, a part of your brain that regulates many of your needs. It, in turn, creates the pulsations or contractions that you feel in your stomach as hunger pangs. Hunger is actually caused by low blood sugar, not by the amount of food you've eaten or how recently you've eaten it. Remain at a low blood-sugar level for too long and you begin to experience fatigue, irritability, and dizziness.

When you place food in your mouth, some of these symptoms go away. Psychologically, the act of chewing—without swallowing—affects the hypothalamus physically. This will not alter your blood-sugar level, however, so food must be put into the stomach.

As you eat, your digestive system begins breaking down the food and sending it through your body. This sends your blood-sugar level back up, giving you more energy. Notice that what counts is not how full your tummy is, but how full of sugar your blood is.

The signal to stop eating

This is the signal your body sends you when you've had enough to eat. You may not have filled your stomach, but you have processed enough food to raise your blood-sugar level, so your body lets you know with subtle changes in your need to obtain food. You'll find yourself slowing down your pace of eating, even if what you're eating is delicious.

Your body is seeking a perfect balance. It knows that it needs certain amounts of food to operate at peak efficiency. You may go on eating past the signal, because you enjoy eating or because you like the taste of the particular food you're having at that moment, but there is no physiological need for that food. By heeding the signal, you can much more easily lose weight and maintain your weight.

What about a craving for candy?

Two things are at work here. First, if your blood-sugar level is low, your body is sending you signals, that you need to eat. Second, you like the taste of candy, so you happily reach for a chocolate bar. The sugar in the candy bar shoots into your bloodstream much faster than almost any other kind of food. (This is why you feel a "lift" after eating chocolate or other candies.)

The problem is that you get so much sugar into your bloodstream in such a short time that your body tries to compensate for it by producing insulin. Insulin is a protein hormone that regulates your metabolism (the ongoing chemical processes in your body relating to your use of food), in this case your metabolism of sugar.

After the insulin lowers your blood-sugar level, your body signals you to eat. You grab a candy bar. Your blood-sugar level rapidly rises, giving you a lift, a boost of energy. Your body produces insulin. The insulin pulls the sugar out of your bloodstream. Your blood-sugar level gets low. And the process repeats.

Except you have added some calories to your body that you cannot burn off right away. And you gain weight. Since the whole process takes about twenty minutes, you can almost predict the changes that come over your body. And, by eating a little or drinking water or juice a half hour before your meals, you'll have started your blood-sugar level back up by the time you sit down for a full meal. This will help you eat less of the meal. It should also help you avoid the sugary foods that actually tend to deplete your energy (in the long run) and that tend to make you want to eat more and more.

Why do you crave other foods?

Your body knows its needs. If you are low in grain, you get a craving for toast, muffins, cereal, and the like. If you are low in protein, you get a craving for eggs, cheese, meat, fish, and so on.

Animals have the same mechanism at work in their bodies. Although this tendency is more pronounced in their wild state, most animals will try to regulate their own intake of foods. Not consciously—we seem to be the creatures who can knowingly react to our body's needs—but with some sort of inner cravings.

When you were three days old, you could tell the difference between a formula based on dextrose (a kind of sugar) and a formula based on milk. We know this because of tests conducted on infants 48 to 90 hours old. The preference, by a wide margin, is for the milk-based formula. Apparently, we are born with the balance-seeking mechanism built in, because all other tests show that we seek to eat foods that will give us a balanced diet in the long run. While you may not eat grain, fruit, vegetable, and protein at every meal, your body will make you find some of each food group sooner or later. If you respect this need for a balanced diet, you can give your body what it needs every single day. This will help you in many ways: fewer tension headaches, fewer bouts of irritability, better regularity, a better complexion, better sleep patterns, and . . . better weight maintenance.

When you are healthy, you can enjoy your meals more. And when you enjoy your meals, you can take the time to control your portions, start your digestion by eating a half hour prior to a full meal, and eat slower—all of which will help you take control of your weight and keep control of it.

Another experiment

Many children under four years of age were given free rein to eat any of several foods presented to them at mealtimes over a period of several days. They all started out sampling the various foods. They all discovered they had one or two favorite foods. For many meals in a row, they chose their favorites. But then, suddenly, they switched their preferences to other foods.

Their bodies began signaling them to add more foods containing different ingredients. It wasn't a matter of taste. After a meal or two in which they provided themselves with the needed foods, they kept on a balanced approach despite showing a preference for their favorite foods.

I mention this experiment to remind you of your own food training when you were young. Your parents did not let you eat just the foods you preferred. They pushed spinach while you hoped for ice cream. So it may be possible that your cravings for some favorite foods when you were a child have been unduly influencing you as an adult. Your parents might have done better letting you have a little more of what you desired, while making certain that you always had access to the other foods. Then, too, they might have done you a disservice in feeding you too much, as we will see.

Sometimes overeating isn't your fault

There is a theory that defines overeating as a compulsive disease, like alcoholism. While this theory does not have the backing of such recognized authoritative bodies as the American Medical Association, it is true that the AMA took quite a long time to recognize alcoholism as a disease, and many of the facts in the cases are similar.

In any event, the theory is worth considering because of similar psychological interpretations in The Ego Diet.

In childhood, your eating patterns helped shape the development of your adipose tissue, or fat cells. Adipose tissue is first formed when you are in the uterus, again during the first two years of life, and once again during early adolescence. So, the more you eat during those periods after birth, the more fat cells you develop. You may have up to five times the number of fat cells as a thin friend. This condition remains constant throughout your life, making it harder for you to lose weight, and easier to gain it.

The average number of fat cells in an average-sized body is somewhere between 30 and 40 billion. But you may have anywhere from 30 to 160 billion fat cells in your body. The more fat cells, the more fat is stored in your body. Cutting down on your food intake may shrink the size of your fat cells, but it will not cut down the number. (This may have been the derivation of the term "reduce" as applied to diet plans.)

The fat cell content theory accounts for part of the reason you may be the same relative size as a friend who eats more than you do. You can eat less than the average person and still not lose weight.

You may have heard the expression "a plump baby is a healthy baby." This used to be true back in the days when more disease was running unchecked in our population. Today, however, the types of diseases parents worried about formerly are not likely to strike a plump baby or an average-sized baby.

It is sad to think that your parents, although well meaning, may have established your body weight disposition in early childhood. Still, this becomes just one more reason why you need to make use of all the psychological techniques available to you in The Ego Diet. Knowing that your weight problem may not be your fault should help you to think better of yourself. Don't get into a funk about it. Just be happy you have discovered you don't lack will power when it comes to eating. Now you know you're not lazy—you're just a little ill. The Ego Diet is your medicine that you can take every day to help you stay well.

WHY YOU GET HUNGRY 109

No fault, but responsibility

Now that you know there is the very real possibility that your weight problems may not be your fault, it is important that you don't use this as an excuse (the old line about wanting to control your desires for candy but being unable to do so). The number of fat cells may not be your fault, but the amount of food you decide to put into your body is still up to you. You can fight your weight or you can give in. I don't believe you're a quitter. You've come this far, haven't you?

Okay, the whole situation—your weight, your eating habits, your having used failure diets (crash diets) in the past—isn't your fault. But despite your being sick with fat cells, it is still your responsibility to do something about your weight. The burden isn't something you can shrug off just because you've got more fat cells than the next person (and perhaps you don't—this hasn't been proved yet).

Facing the responsibility

This should be a healthy experience. You may come out of it feeling much better today than you did yesterday. Tomorrow you may feel better still.

All the doubts about yourself can now just go away. You know you're going to have more self-respect. More self-esteem. More confidence. How? Because you have taken the time to think through your situation. You've put in the effort of reading about yourself in this book. You've nodded in agreement, shook your head in dismay, and made notes of ideas you want to try. You're already moving in the right direction. For crying out loud, how many other people even bother to find out what makes them get hungry in the first place?

Hold your head up high. (There—that alone, just standing up straight, takes five pounds off your figure.)

Can digestion itself make you hungry?

It shouldn't, but it depends on what you eat. If you were to eat only sugar, but very slowly, you might be able to go through a low blood-sugar/high blood-sugar/low blood-sugar cycle while still eating. In other words, your digestive process may contribute to a situation in which you keep getting hungry. This is only a hypothetical situation, however (or at least I hope it is never a reality for someone).

Is there such a thing as sugar addiction?

That depends on who is defining the terms involved. Technically, you are addicted to something if you go through withdrawal upon its removal. If you want a certain substance, whether it is food, drink, or drugs, and you begin to suffer physically or psychologically when you cannot have it, then you are addicted to that substance. In this sense, yes, there is such a thing as addiction to sugar. Your body craves the "jag" or lift you get from the rise in your blood-sugar level. Your mind associates well-being with the rise in excess energy that accompanies the jag.

The odds are that you are not addicted to sugar. You merely find it tasty, as millions of us do. If you think that you are addicted to sugar, see your doctor.

Here's a quick test to determine your level of attraction (let's call it that, shall we?) to sugar. Think about this choice: you cannot have any sugar unless you visit your doctor to have a series of blood tests, a stomach pump inserted down your throat, or a gloved finger inserted up your rectum. Now, how do you feel about it? If you were addicted, you'd either know that none of these things would be too horrible a price to pay, or you'd have already tossed this book aside in disgust at my forcing you to confront such a choice. The normal, healthy person does not volunteer for any of the hospital procedures outlined above unless a real gain may come from them; the gain usually is the diagnosis of an illness or the prevention of one.

Will my taste buds make me hungry?

Your taste buds, which are located on your tongue and other parts of your mouth, do nothing to contribute to your sense of hunger. Your mind makes you recall the sensation of tasting certain foods, causing you to salivate. You might think about the taste of something and in so doing you might think you are tasting it. More common is the feeling that a certain taste is just out of reach. This leads to the sometimes obsessive behavior usually associated with alcoholics—searching the cupboards for a certain kind of food, driving from one store to another to find it, and so forth.

You can easily and quickly control the sensation of tasting something that isn't there just by putting something there. Eat a cracker, drink some water or juice, or chew some gum. This will give you time to become distracted by some other interest.

Another trick you might want to try is this: think of a food that has the opposite taste of whatever it is that you're imagining. If, for example, you're convinced that the taste of a juicy dill pickle is "just on the tip of your tongue," and you feel you shan't rest until your taste buds are satisfied, deliberately force yourself to think about the taste of a nice, cold glass of milk. If, after that, the craving for the pickle returns, you have to decide if your body could possibly be telling you something. Perhaps you have too severely restricted your intake of salt. It may not be the pickle itself that you need or want, but what's in the pickle.

Can foods themselves make me hungry?

No, your body controls your hunger for certain foods. Or rather, for what's in certain foods. There are two general classifications of food. There are inorganic foods, such as salt and water. And there are organic foods, like carbohydrates, proteins, fats, and vitamins.

When you eat certain foods, your body breaks them down, uses part of them for energy and part of them to repair worn out tissue or parts of organs. The foods you eat are also used to promote the flexibility and contractibility of muscles and the conductivity of your nervous system tissues.

The breaking down of food is accomplished automatically. Enzymes (proteins created in your body by cells) are able to speed up the chemical processes that take place inside you. The fact that your body secretes the right enzymes for each kind of food is in itself a miracle of life. There must be a balance of acidity and alkalinity in addition to all the other problems of digestion. And the building blocks from the broken down foodstuffs must be transported to various parts of your body in order to perform their work.

That's when the other cells in your body extract what they need from the food passing through your blood. Some goes into keeping your blood-sugar level normal. Some is used to keep your body warm. Some is stored so as to be available later to maintain that blood-sugar level (it keeps coming back, doesn't it?).

When you eat too much, it gets stored as adipose tissue, or fat.

Let's say you eat well. That is, you choose foods from the four basic food groups: grain, meat, milk, fruit and vegetable. Through the process of digestion, protein and fat from any source can be turned into fuel for your body. What you eat during the day becomes heat, water, carbon dioxide, and waste material (which is simply the product of all the effort of extraction of the "good stuff" in the food). If only all the "bad stuff" you ate would turn into waste material. It doesn't. It goes to your hips. Or tummy. Or . . . you know best where it affects you.

Whatever you need in your body, whether it is material to repair some minor damage to your liver or just more energy to face a meeting the next day, your body will signal you by making you hungry for foods that contain the necessary ingredients. The trick is in not confusing your desire for instant taste gratification with the very real need for specific nutrients in specific foods.

Common sense is going to help you through this problem. If you find yourself craving a dish of ice cream, don't just assume that your body needs something in the ice cream. Stop and ask yourself what that "something" might be. After a moment of thought, it will be obvious that you don't need the ice cream, but the dairy product on which it's based. You weren't giving your body enough milk, so you got a subtle signal to drink some. You missed the signal. So your body simply escalated the signals. You got the message this time, but you garbled it. Your body wants dairy products, not ice cream. You like the taste of ice cream, so you conveniently confused the craving for milk with your craving for the taste of the sweeter ice cream.

Think it through

Consider your body's needs and it will treat you right. When you think about eating something, ask yourself what's in the food. You know that a hot dog is not as healthy for you as a piece of baked fish or fresh fish in sushi. You might still decide to have the hot dog, but you must at least consider the fat content, the additives, the chemical preservatives, and the oil in many of the things associated with eating hot dogs (onions, for instance).

All that The Ego Diet requires is for you to think through the consequences of eating any food. Is it good for you? Will it help your digestion? Will it interfere with your sleep?

Only then do you get to ask yourself that all-important question, the one that used to be the determining factor in all your eating decisions: does it taste good?

12

Why Most Diets Fail

MOST diets fail because they never get started. Of those that do get started, most fail because . . . well, what were the reasons in your case?

Excuses, excuses

There are tons of reasons for not sticking to a healthy diet plan. Let's look at a few of them. Some will sound familiar to you. You've heard your friends use them. You've used them yourself.

> "I don't really need to lose weight, I just need some toning up."

> "I skipped lunch today, so it's okay to eat a big meal now."

> "It's all right to eat more, because everyone always gains weight on vacation."

> "Having big portions is not going to hurt, because Chinese food is mainly vegetables."

> "Yeah, I'm eating a lot now, but I'll fast tomorrow."

> "I'm not having any garlic bread, so I can have another plate of spaghetti."

You can probably list a few more common rationalizations that signify that a person isn't sticking to a good diet. The underlying fact in all of these excuses is this: the speaker wants his or her cake and to lose weight, too. Sure, you might be able to burn off some extra calories if you're about to engage in some unusually athletic endeavor, but that is precisely the wrong time to indulge in heavy foods like pasta or to over-eat because it tastes good.

The argument about not having to lose weight because some toning up is needed carries no weight, so to speak, because people who don't need to lose weight don't have to announce it. And if you could look good with a little toning up, what are you waiting for? Get moving to the next chapter and begin the toning process.

The reasoning that you can go berserk at the dinner table because you skipped lunch is spotty, at best. Skipping lunch has nothing to do with being able to add food to your regular meal portions. That's a good way to stuff your stomach to the point where you cause yourself pain. And eating extra at one meal to make up the difference between the current meal and the one you skipped forces your body to digest more food at one time than it can handle. So what does your body do with the excess food? It converts the food to adipose tissue for later or forever, depending on your subsequent behavior.

People who use a vacation as a reason to pig out are like people who use a party as a reason to get stinking drunk. Sure, there's a difference in degree, but not in kind.

Big portions of food are big portions of food. If you ate enough lettuce you'd get fat.

Saying you'll fast tomorrow to make up for today is both foolhardy and a lie. It is much healthier to spread out 4,000 calories over two days than to have 3,000 one day and zero the next. Besides, how many people actually do fast the next day?

Saying that you'll have one extra helping of a heavy food because you're passing up an extra helping of some other heavy food is akin to being proud that you didn't smash up your car's right fender right after you just crumpled the left one. If you're eating too much, you're eating too much—it doesn't matter what or how you do it.

The case for fat

One big problem with people in Western culture has to do with our popular media: television, movies, and pulp fiction. Usually there are clear-cut lines drawn between right and wrong, good and evil, hero and villain. So when it comes to a diet, it is easy to cast all fats as the evil, snarling villain. Your body needs fats and fat-related substances. They are an energy source that can be stored up and used as needed throughout the day. And you need a layer of body fat to provide insulation against cold (or rather, against loss of body heat).

Since your body will demand some fats by making you crave foods with high fat content, you'll do one of two things. You'll fight against the healthy and normal instincts of your own body, causing anxiety and distress. Or you'll give in and may blame yourself for lacking the strength to combat what you mistakenly believe is an evil desire.

Then, too, there's the fact that your own perfect weight may not be the same as that of a fashion model your size. This is almost the reverse of hating fat, in that it can become an excuse to ignore your ego needs for maintaining your weight rather than gaining. There is no denying that people can be attractive at various sizes and shapes. Goodness knows we don't always insist that our friends have the same color hair, eyes, clothing, whatever; so perhaps it is healthy to accept people— including ourselves—even if a bit overweight by our standards.

This in no way condones people who are flabby, out of shape, or grossly obese. But these conditions shouldn't be confused with pleasantly plump and zaftig. If you see your doctor and find out that your heart rate, blood pressure, cholesterol, and normal bodily functions are in good shape, then I say you're in good shape no matter what your body looks like. If you feel good at your current weight, then use this book to maintain your weight. This diet plan will fail if you're already at your ideal weight and shape and you try to force yourself to lose.

Most people want to lose weight, then maintain it

Face it: most of us want to lose a few pounds before going on a weight-maintenance program.

While it is certainly true that no amount of good advice about healthy dieting will do any good if the advice isn't followed, it is also true that the right psychological approach can make sure the advice *can be followed.* The first step in this chapter has already been taken: an understanding of the excuse syndrome. The next step is an examination of the many outside factors that cause diet plans to go awry.

What if you're cynical about all diets?

That's a reason for avoiding a healthy diet in the first place, but it isn't a reason for giving up on one once you've accepted it. Because The Ego Diet works from within you, any cynicism you may have built up toward all other diet plans should be fairly easily dissipated. In fact, the greater the cynicism, the healthier the ego; therefore, the better you'll be on The Ego Diet.

The boredom factor

As you know, many other diet plans tell you what to eat at every meal for weeks on end. This rigidity leads to boredom with the diet.

Even if you can put up with that, because other diets don't give you anything to work with psychologically, you have to try to boost yourself by constantly talking about your diet. This bores your friends before it bores you, but it does bore even you after a while.

Overeating is often an antidote to boredom in your life. People who've had a change of job, where they've gone from doing something interesting to performing mundane tasks, frequently eat on the job. This can be a particularly vexing problem if you have the kind of job that alternates between periods of activity and periods with lots of downtime.

One friend of mine went through this problem for two years before finding a cure. During her job's dull moments, she removes the covers from technical magazines in her field of business, places them over other magazines that she likes to read, and buries herself in pleasurable reading.

While this may not be practical for you, it is possible to combat the boredom in ways that won't cause you to give up your diet plan. Think about what kinds of mental activity will keep you sharp during the day.

One lady executive I know says she always seems to have a dead spot in the late afternoon when there are no calls to make, no meetings to attend, and no more paperwork left to wade through. She used to snack her way through the rest of the day. Now, she says she mentally reviews every conversation she had during the day to make notes of important bits of information she might otherwise forget, or to reflect on how she might have handled a decision better. "You'd be surprised," she confided in me, "how often a business deal seems to depend on being able to remember some otherwise insignificant detail—a detail that I may have made note of only during one of my 'reverie' sessions." And, of course, she doesn't add pounds to her body, either. This is a great combination: a weight maintenance method that makes you better in business. She has found a way to use boredom in a creative way . . . and thus never be bored.

Trouble with your marriage

Some diets fail because your spouse doesn't support you in your efforts. It's pretty hard to concentrate on the good, healthy foods when your partner brings home a bucket of fried chicken every night. This is just a matter of basic communication. Make your feelings known and frankly ask for help and consideration.

There is another problem that can develop into a real diet breaker. If you're not getting enough love and attention from your mate, you might be going on a perpetual-failure diet. That is, if you get attention

—sympathy, mainly, but attention nevertheless—because of your struggles to diet, then you'll do whatever you can to keep on getting the attention. Having trouble with your diet is what gets you the attention, so you automatically do things that cause you to have trouble. You fail to lose weight. What is odd about situations like this is that the lack of attention in the first place might stem from your being overweight.

Don't be worried about your weight. Conscientious, yes. But not worried. And don't be obsessed with the foods you've already eaten. Because if you're sitting there brooding about the French fries you had for lunch, chances are you're not thinking about your lover. Or thinking about making love with your lover. Or actually making love . . . well, you get the picture.

Getting stuck at one weight level

Whether or not you use the scales, you still can tell if you aren't reducing. At least you can tell over a long enough period of time. Many people become discouraged when their weight doesn't change and they begin to reprimand themselves. Don't you dare. Be happy you didn't gain any weight. All your efforts at eating healthy foods are paying off because you're not ballooning up in size the way you would if you hadn't done all that work.

A great many people are incapable of turning what they consider a bad situation—not losing weight—into a good and positive thing, namely that they're not gaining any weight. Don't get caught in this trap. You know whether you've been eating according to a healthy diet plan, so you know whether you should redouble your efforts to follow one of the Ego Diet methods in this book. I say, if you get to the weight that makes you feel comfortable, if your doctor agrees you're in good physical shape, and if you're able to stay on your diet plan with ease— then you're one of the fortunate people who has found an ideal weight . . . no matter what some chart may tell you about recommended weight for your height.

Those damn charts

You've probably gazed forlornly at one of the countless height/weight charts showing your recommended weight five or ten pounds below where you are at the moment (or even five to ten pounds below the weight you hope to reach in a few months).

You look at your weight and discover that you should be two or three inches taller to make the table's "desirable weight." Your eye sways over to the classification marked "large frame" or "big boned." Aha! You're at the proper weight in this column. But how many of us have the skeletal system of a tag-team wrestler? Come on, you're not "big boned," not really. Or are you?

That's the rub. What in tarnation is "small framed"? Or "medium boned"? Nobody has ever defined these terms, so it's impossible to tell what these charts are telling us. Do yourself a favor and toss them in the circular file. Rely on the pinch procedure. Or the mirror method. Or just go by the way you feel.

A negative attitude

If you get down on yourself for even having to control your diet, you'll never succeed. No matter the reason for your negative feelings, they will not help you on your healthy diet plan. The psychological stress this adds to your life can lead to both mental and physical fatigue. The anxiety you experience over negative feelings regarding your self-worth can aggravate a heart condition. So keep this in mind: You are so important a person in the world (or at least in your part of the world) that you must take control of your eating habits. That's not a bad thing, it's a good thing. Being on The Ego Diet is a positive sign. It's a signal that you and your health are worth taking time and effort to protect— right, protect. Only someone who is crucial in his or her job would need a psychological diet-reinforcement plan as sophisticated as The Ego Diet.

So buck up. You're worth fussing over.

Illness

Some diets are unhealthy. Crash diets especially. They can take all the minerals out of you along with all the calories. If your system has nothing with which to fight off disease, you're going to get sick.

Women need iron, for example, and it's better to get it in your food than in a pill. If you cut out the wrong foods because you're busy cutting out all foods, you can shortchange yourself.

If you get sick during a crash diet, you have to restock your body with whatever the diet has denied you. In so doing, you might tend to eat the wrong foods and fall off your diet as you regain your health. This can certainly be true of colds, when you find yourself constantly raiding the refrigerator, always seeking to have something to chew and swallow. Part of the reason for this has to do with the soothing feeling food has on your throat. It also keeps your mind off the stuffiness in your nasal passages.

Let me put the clincher to you—you are less likely to get ill with a healthy diet plan like The Ego Diet.

Sabotage

Beware the jealous friend. You'll be admired for sticking to your diet, but you'll also be a target for those who are upset by your success. They may disguise their jealousy by joking with you or teasing you, but the words sound exactly the same no matter what the tone of voice:

"Oh come on, have a piece of pie. You can always diet tomorrow."

They may keep up this line of talk over a long period of time, so be prepared to smile while shaking your head "no." If you don't like hearing a constant urging to eat foods you know are wrong for you, speak up about it. You don't have to get mad about it, just state nicely but firmly that you know what's right for you and that your refusal to indulge in no way reflects on anyone else's choice of food. Then change the subject. Perhaps you can turn the tables on them by complimenting them on the way they look.

Sometimes the jealousy manifests itself in ridicule:

"Oh, here comes the person with the big ego . . . and the big belly."

There is never any good response to an adult who acts like a child. All you can do is say, in as philosophical a tone as you can manage, that the person is being childish, and exit the room. Don't get into a shouting match about it or feel you have to stand there and put yourself on such a person's level.

Parents

We've already seen how parents, even with the best of intentions, can spoil a good diet plan. A government-funded study of nearly a quarter of a million dieters found that mothers may sometimes view a child's diet as a form of rejection, even if her child is fully grown and living away from home. Feeding her baby was so important a task, and so filled with love, that food and love get intermingled in the mother's mind. By going on a diet, you are seemingly rejecting some of your mother's love.

When your mom tries to get you to eat more, tell her you love her. Then say no to the food. It'll work.

Moods

If you get satisfaction from eating and your diet takes this satisfaction away, then you're left with a minor form of anxiety that can only be called moodiness. It's a feeling of having been prevented from doing something. You feel thwarted, pent up, frustrated.

This is enough for many people to break off their diets. It certainly was enough for me before The Ego Diet. Now, because of the elegant, leisurely dining recommended by The Ego Diet, I still get quite a bit of pleasure out of mealtime (even if I don't get the same amount of food as before).

If you can be relaxed when eating, you'll be halfway toward being satisfied with slightly smaller portions and a slight changeover from rich foods to healthier ones.

Failure built in from the start

What did you do in high school, go out on dates or find excuses for staying home? If you dated, you can skip this section. If you stayed home too much, read on.

Were dates out of reach because you were shy? Timid? Just plain scared? Did you cover up your feelings by finding other things to do—like eat? A lot of people do. When you should have been socializing, you were snacking. Instead of nibbling on someone's ear you were nibbling on a candy bar.

This may be why you are having trouble with most other diet plans. You didn't gain any satisfaction from the opposite sex, but you did gain a lot of pleasure from food. And now, you're stuck with food as your own private pleasure principle.

You may not even need a diet. Find something you enjoy doing, and get involved. Be it hobby or avocation, if it brings you pleasure and doesn't involve food, do it and do it regularly. See what happens after several weeks have gone by. You might be happy to know that being happier leads to a lessening of a weight problem.

What about the word "diet"?

Okay, it's an ugly word. It doesn't sound nice. (Oddly enough, despite having the sound of death in its first syllable, it actually comes from a Greek term meaning "way of life.")

You may not want to admit you're on a diet, even one as powerful-sounding as The Ego Diet. While I think that you should feel free to use the word diet in its true sense—your intake of food, or your food plan

—you certainly can use The Ego Diet and not tell anyone about it. If this helps you, great.

Diet doesn't have to refer to food. Think of it as relating to your behavior as a whole. The way you dress, hold yourself, and the way you move are all part of your diet. The way you trim your hair is also a part of it.

Diet, or at least The Ego Diet, encompasses everything you do that relates to your health and well-being, to a healthy "way of life." By keeping that in mind, you should find the term more friendly.

Fat as protection

Some people use their bulk as a defense mechanism against the world. They consider it armor. If this is the case, reducing weight represents a threat because it means giving up their fleshy form of protection. The more successful the reducing scheme, the more they reject it. This isn't necessarily a conscious decision on their part, which is why this situation is very difficult to deal with. How do you convince such individuals that their excess weight is a defeatist way to deal with the world, especially when they are so comfortable with their security blanket of flesh?

You don't. Direct confrontation is just what they've been avoiding by eating their way inside a human buffer zone. The only thing that works is showing them they are good people, with value, intelligence, and strength . . . and that these things are a part of them no matter what they weigh. And, since they'll be around longer without the excess weight, why not encourage them to lose just a bit of it? One day at a time.

"It makes me weak"

If you work hard all day, whether it's at physical or mental tasks, you'll feel fatigued at night. If you haven't done much during the day, but still feel tired and listless, you have false fatigue.

This feeling often overtakes people who are just starting diet plans, especially ones that attempt too large a cutback in food. The feeling becomes an excellent excuse for giving up on the good intentions of the diet plan.

If this problem of false fatigue hits you, day or night, be sure you muster all your strength and . . . take it sitting down. Really, you don't have to battle this feeling. Just stop what you're doing and rest for a couple of minutes. All that's happening is your body is adjusting to the new feeding schedule you've established. After five minutes have passed, get up slowly, stretch your arms toward the ceiling, and go back to your work or play.

Loneliness

Being lonely is terrible. Everyone wants and needs the friendship and companionship of others. And everyone goes through periods when others are not available: the wife whose husband goes away on business; the husband whose wife gets involved in a career of her own; the "new kid in town"—anyone who has changed jobs, moved, or gone through the breakup of a relationship knows what this phrase means. All these situations lead to feeling lonely.

When loneliness sets in, it's tempting to assuage it by eating. This goes back to the satisfaction, comfort, and security you felt as a baby whenever you were fed. To regain that good feeling and cast off the feeling of being cast off, you can either eat good foods or bad foods. I hope you choose good foods. I also hope you put on your most comfortable outfit and go out somewhere. Go where there is dancing, laughter, excitement. Go to a movie. Go bowling. Just move it on out to something that interests you. Chances are you'll meet someone who is feeling the same way, and you can talk about that to start things going.

It is a cliché of situation comedies on television that some bars are warm and friendly places where wonderful and joyous events regularly take place. I have been in only two or three places where the bar could in any way be called warm and friendly. Crowded and raucous is more like it. Still, if you find a bar in your neighborhood that has a good atmosphere, by all means patronize it. You don't have to swill drinks all night long in order to drop in and chat. You don't even have to order alcoholic beverages.

Guilt

A child of overly strict parents will feel resentment toward his or her father and mother. These feelings will, in turn, lead to guilt feelings. Even when justifiable, anger directed at one's parents is an emotional minefield.

To resolve the guilt feelings, some people will punish themselves, and some do it by overeating to make themselves fat and unattractive.

The above example is only one of dozens of classic cases that have been duplicated over and over again for years. The basic point about unhealthy eating habits being a form of self-punishment holds true for a great many of these cases. If this is a serious problem for you, seeing a psychologist might be a good idea.

If this seems like something you can handle on your own, you might take a few minutes each day to think about your relationship with your parents, both now and when you were young. See if you can find any link between your feelings and the way you now eat. Often, just considering the problem makes it much easier to deal with and the ability to stay with a healthy diet is greatly improved.

13

Move It!

FOOD is energy. Just like putting gasoline into your car, eating is a way of filling up with fuel. The more you put in, the farther you can go. Or, what is more to the point, the more you put in, the farther you'd better go—or you risk gaining weight.

Food isn't in the right form for your body to use, so a series of chemical and physical processes—metabolism—breaks it down to provide energy for all your life activities. It takes a certain number of calories each day to meet your particular metabolic needs. It is in this area that the use of the word calorie is most proper, because a calorie is really a scientific measurement of energy (there are about 4,000 calories in each pound of fat in your body).

Not counting elimination, there are only two things that can happen to the food you put into your body. First, you can use it for fuel to keep your body going. This includes all the vital functions such as the operation of your heart, lungs, organs, nervous system, and so forth, as well as your muscles.

Second, you can store the excess food on your body and carry it around with you as—you guessed it—fat.

Bear in mind that your body uses up calories even while you're resting; even while you're asleep. Each of us has what is known as a Resting Metabolic Rate, which is the minimum number of calories needed to maintain your vital functions each day. The RMR varies depending on your body size, age, and weight. So it can be 1,200 calories a day for someone weighing 115 pounds and 1,800 calories a day for a 180-pounder.

As for the amount of food that winds up exiting your body as waste material, well, that's only significant when you're having trouble getting rid of it. Otherwise, the body is a very efficient machine. Few, if any, calories are ever lost.

The amount of energy you take in must be equaled by the amount of energy you put out. If you eat 4,000 calories but only burn off 3,000, you just gained a quarter of a pound of fat.

Take in more than you put out and you gain weight; put out more than you take in and you lose weight. That's where the "putting out" part comes in. It's called exercise.

You need it

You need to move your body. Even bedridden patients are given exercise programs. Hospital studies of bedridden people of all ages reveal that the weight, density, and strength of a patient's bones decreases. The decrease occurs for as long as the patient remains motionless. This critical loss of bone mass is accomplished in a relatively short time. What this means to you may be gathered by a glance at the insurance company tables concerning broken bones by age of victim. Ask your life insurance agent to show you this sometime. The accidents that would be just a bump to you are literal bone breakers for senior citizens.

In this country, older people very often have weak, brittle bones, making them highly susceptible to fractures. Even in jolts that would be quite minor if their bone mass was at a normal level, elderly people can suffer debilitating injuries. The reasons for this are becoming clearer to researchers all over the globe. Our sedentary life-style is the culprit. Too little physical activity is contributing to much pain and suffering, all of which could so easily be avoided.

Live longer

The populations of three places in the world are noted for having an unusually high proportion of people who live beyond the age of 100 years. The three areas are the Ecuadorian mountains, the Himalayas, and a region in the Soviet Union called Georgia. The life-style in these areas is rugged by our standards, with much of the populace engaged in farming.

Despite their diet being much lower than ours in calcium, their bones are quite well calcified and strong. Apparently the physical activity which is a part of their daily routine has helped keep their skeletal systems strong. This, in turn, has kept them more willing and able to maintain a healthy, vigorous, and active life. And both factors have evidently contributed to their longevity.

So the old jive saying, "you got to move it not to lose it," is true. The documentation concerning lowered bone mass being a result of inactivity extends even to our astronaut program. In the weightlessness of space—where you don't need as much muscle action to propel your body—our astronauts have experienced a 7 percent loss of bone mass in just a few weeks of orbiting the earth. One could even make a case for inactivity being an accelerated aging process.

You'll eat less

It may not sound possible, but test after test has shown that people tend to slightly decrease their intake of food when a moderate exercise program is started. Notice I said *moderate* exercise program. There is no need to overdo it, as you'll soon see.

Your entire system of body functions, including eating, can be thrown into disarray by a lack of exercise. The appetite center of your brain, the hypothalamus, does not work properly when physical activity is curtailed. If you are forced to remain relatively motionless, the signals from the hypothalamus to your body will become garbled.

Also important is the fact that the body's signals to stop eating are equally affected by a lack of exercise. The act of eating is usually continued far too long by inactive people. They take in more food than is required for the small amount of activity their bodies go through. Then, their bodies have no choice but to store the excess as fat. This may be useful if you intend to become stranded on a desert island but is otherwise not recommended.

Two groups of people were tested during a controlled weight-loss program. One group was allowed to remain sedentary, but the other was led through a relatively minor exercise program. Both groups lost weight, but there were two crucial differences between them.

First, the people who did not exercise were slightly dehydrated. Fifty percent of the weight they lost was either water or protein. This they gained back almost as soon as they returned to their normal eating patterns. But the group that performed a few exercises did much better. Only a quarter of the weight they lost was water or protein. Seventy-five percent of the weight they lost was fat.

Second, the people in the exercise group who continued their exercise program (but not the weight-loss program) were able to maintain their new, lower weight.

Your "stomach clock"

In one of the *Peanuts* cartoon strips, Snoopy the beagle brings his supper dish up to Charlie Brown, who then tells Snoopy to go back to his doghouse because it isn't yet time for supper. Snoopy looks out of the next picture in a puzzled manner and says to himself, "My stomach clock must be fast."

Your body sends you signals when it's time to eat. It also signals you the right kinds of things to eat. If you need fuel, you'll feel it. Usually it's because your appetite is aroused. Other times, you begin to get a headache that never seems to get bad enough to require the aspirin. Or you may find yourself getting tense and irritable for no reason. All these are signals that you need to send your body some good, healthy food.

But if you're not moving your body during the day, these signals don't occur at the right time. Your stomach clock goes off or on at random times. Why? Scientists and doctors believe it is because we aren't getting enough exercise, which is the direct result of too much being done for us.

The percentage of people in our society performing physical labor for a living is steadily decreasing. We have machines to do our laundry, dishes, food preparation, and more. We have bigger machines to transport us from place to place. When was the last time you beat your laundry clean on a rock? Or even just walked to the store instead of driving?

All right, I can hear you protesting that the stores are several miles from your house and you couldn't possibly carry five bags of groceries home from there. I agree. I'm not suggesting that you're lazy because you take the car to the store. The point is that our lives are designed to rely on machines and not on our bodies. I mean, elevators and escalators take us where stairs used to, even when we finally reach the stores.

Consider the old ticker

A twenty-year study by the American Cancer Society demonstrated that people who keep up even a slight amount of regular exercise are far less likely to suffer from stroke or coronary heart disease.

Look what can happen to your heart with just a small amount of overeating. Let's say you begin eating just one extra food item each day, a small item like a cup of fruit yogurt. This is adding about 250 calories to the amount of extra food you may already take in—that is, the amount over and above what you need to balance your energy needs. In a month, you would have gained about three pounds.

Keep this up month after month, year after year, and your heart has to do more work just to maintain a normal blood flow. If you also avoid physical activity whenever possible, you are robbing your heart of a chance to build up its muscular strength, which is different from its strength as a regulator of fluid. You begin to have a less and less efficient pumping action, so the heart speeds up some more. And the more it speeds up, the less reserve capacity you have.

And the closer you are to a heart attack.

Predicting who will keep weight off

In a weight-loss program conducted at the University of Southern California, research psychologist Albert R. Marston was able to predict who among the forty-seven participants would maintain their new, lower weight. His accuracy was 90 percent, based on a questionnaire that was completed before the weight-loss program was administered.

Marston said that two factors contributed to the success of the "maintainers." The first was emotional stability. Those who did not eat for psychological reasons were more likely to be able to maintain their weight. The second, and more important, was the maintenance of a regular exercise program.

Marston noted that "The maintainers who exercised several times a week . . . had the best chance of avoiding relapses. Lack of exercise seemed to be a crucial factor among the relapse group."

Better sleep habits

You'll sleep better and feel more refreshed if you perform even a few exercises each day. There may even be a connection between lack of exercise, poor eating habits, and the inability to fall asleep easily and/or sleep soundly.

Upon awakening, you will find that your whole morning doesn't have to be shrouded in a fog of befuddlement if you'll just move your body for a couple of minutes of exercise.

Pleasure (sometimes)

Regular exercise, even if confined to 340 seconds a day, will help your posture, clear your head, strengthen your heart, improve your complexion, cut your appetite, ease feelings of anxiety, bolster your circulation, and lift you out of depression. And every now and then, it's pleasurable.

I admit that four or five days a week I just go through my exercises by rote, with little pleasure taken at the precise moment I'm exercising. If I skip my routine, however, I don't feel perky, my back aches, and I generally feel as if I've just been turned down for a job and found a parking ticket on my car. And the knowledge that that is what awaits me if I don't get a move on each morning keeps me going through the motions.

Two or three times a week, a magical thing happens. I begin to feel the power of my muscles and I get mentally involved with my physical activities. It is exhilarating when that occurs, and the "high" continues throughout the morning. Sometimes it even continues through the entire day, but this is, I admit, rather dependent on how the day goes; if I'm forced to deal with bozos and bozoettes every other minute, it's difficult to remain convinced that all is right with the world. Still, the exercising gets me off to a good start, and that's worth a great deal.

Tone

Muscle tone is a firmness and fitness that everyone can see and some can (if they're lucky or you're not careful) touch. If you have good muscle tone, your flesh will not sag as much due to age, so you'll look younger longer.

Since muscle is more compact than fat, you may fit into those tight clothes even if you remain at the same weight after starting your own regular exercise plan. And, since muscle weighs more than flab, you'll be able to keep a feeling of power and size even though you lose some weight. Either way, you win.

Role models

Some people find they can motivate themselves to keep on their exercise program by thinking about a role model. If you admire some well-known person in the media or in sports, and you discover that thinking of him or her gets you to move through your routine, then by all means plaster photos of this person on your wall or refrigerator.

It may be even better to consider those things you have in common with your role model and imagine yourself as you'll look after sticking with your exercise program for a while. Imagine yourself talking with— or better, exercising with—your role model.

Remember that you already have one thing in common with your role model: you're both on an exercise and diet program. Every sports figure and everyone with an image to maintain must also maintain his or her weight. So think of yourself as one of these elite people while you move it. After all, in your own field of endeavor, *you are one of the elite.* So act like it.

Walking

One of the best exercises in the world is also one of the most civilized: walking. Or, as some of us like to refer to it, slow jogging.

Some cities only reveal their full beauty to the walker. Even such antiwalker metropolises as Los Angeles have many areas that are most pleasant for a stroll.

Walks are perfect for quiet contemplation or intimate conversation, but they are even quite pleasing when you're simply trying to get from one place to another when on an errand.

Go for a stroll anytime the inclination strikes you. It is exercise that only requires good shoes. You may not even notice that it's helping your heart, arms, legs, lungs, and circulation. Walking is one of the most painless exercises known.

Jogging

At the risk of offending millions of probably healthy individuals, I must admit I don't care for jogging. I've got nothing against it, you understand. It is a very good form of exercise, and if it appeals to you, great. It's just not for me.

I can't stand the pain. Back pain, mainly, although foot pains have also bothered me. The constant bouncing sends a jolt along my spine that aggravates an old injury I sustained in a traffic accident a decade ago.

It may be sour grapes, then, that makes me list these other objections to jogging: irate dogs, and what they tend to leave deposited on the trails; car and bus exhaust; the stupid outfits you wind up wearing; shinsplints; and, for women, irritated nipples.

Still, if jogging is the exercise that gets you up and about, more power to you. It is so important to keep up a bit of movement each day that I'd recommend anything short of jumping off cliffs. You may have been effectively neglecting your body for the past quarter of a century, but after just a couple of weeks of daily exercise you'll already be reversing the sagging, drooping, and double rolling of your flesh. It is actually quite impressive that the human body is so responsive. And it's lucky for you this is so, assuming you were anything like I was when it came to exercise. I had to be forced into it. Now, however, I embrace it.

Fool yourself

Park your car at the other end of the lot. Find a reason for doing it besides giving you a bit of a walk. Perhaps you can park without cars on either side of your car, thus protecting the sides from other people bashing their doors into yours. Maybe there's some shade to keep your steering wheel and dashboard from baking to cracking temperature by the sun. Possibly you'll be nearer a security guard or a busy street so that there'll be less chance of someone breaking into your car.

Whatever the reason, use that if you can't face the fact that you need to force yourself to take a walk. You may find other benefits besides doing your body some good. One man told me he refused an executive-level parking space on the grounds that he wanted his car facing away from the afternoon sun. The workers he supervised thought they had at last found a supervisor who was "one of them," and they pushed his department's productivity to an all-time high.

I always try to drive at least four blocks past my next destination in hopes of finding a parking space in which I can park for free or for a few coins (instead of the ransom-level fees the commercial parking lots are demanding these days). Sometimes I get the cheap spot. Plus a little exercise.

Sure, in the rain it is a different matter. Then I try to get the best—that is, driest—spot. But I know, if I'm forced to take a hike through the storm, that I'm in better shape to do it than I otherwise would have been.

Fooling yourself as to your real reason for walking is only necessary for compulsive exercise-avoiders and people who live in Los Angeles. All others, just put one foot in front of the other and keep on walking to better health.

Exercise your anger

You can sometimes combine two healthy activities when you find yourself filled with anger and frustration over the events of your life. This situation happens every couple of weeks for me, and almost everyone I talk to admits there are times when he or she just wants to scream and hit something.

When this happens to you, take advantage of it. Get some good, clean, sweaty activity going and stay with it a while. What's that? You say that's not your thing? Oh come on, go shoot some baskets, swim a few laps, pump some iron, bicycle a few miles. No? Well, okay. I don't do those things, either.

What I do is act out what I really would like to do. I hit something. Hard. Many times. While shouting at the top of my lungs.

Before you become repulsed by this blatant display of gratuitous violence, I should point out that the object of my disaffection is the mattress on my bed and old pillow.

I get out the tired and ratty pillow, place it on the edge of the bed down at the footboard, and give it a couple of backhand slaps, just to get warmed up. Then I graduate to pokes, jabs, whaps, whumps, until I give in to the sheer joy of full-bore, arms-flailing-like-windmills assault.

I find that yelling to beat the band just adds to the relief I feel later on when the outburst is over, so I scream the most fearsome swearwords I know over and over again to rid my system of them. If you can't bring yourself to swear, shout some condescending commands—things you'd like to say to your boss, for example, like "Wise up, sucker!" or "Behave like a man, turkey!" A very sweet, devoutly Christian young lady I know told me her favorite phrase was "Eat . . ." Well, perhaps discretion is the better part of valor. Still, you get the point: you can perform this stunt in privacy and emerge a saner, better individual for it. Don't be afraid to let all your anger come flowing out of your guts. You'll get your heart pumping, your arms moving, and your private demons exorcised at the same time. And you'll feel better for it.

The "Gerry Larry" minimum daily requirement of exercise

I am Gerry Larry. Gerry for Gerald, Larry for Laurence. And here's what I do every morning (with a few alternate moves tossed in for you to play around with).

You already know about "the stretch," where you try to touch the sky. I begin with one of those.

Next, stand up straight, feet flat on the floor, arms held straight out from the shoulders so you're forming a cross in the air. Move your arms backward, as though you were going to touch the backs of your hands together behind your back. You'll never even come close to touching your hands, of course (unless you're double-jointed somewhere), but the stretching of your muscles is good for you anyway. Go up on your toes as you do three movements of your arms—back, back, back—then go back down on your heels for the fourth movement, which involves bending your arms at the elbows and then sending your elbows back until your fists are even with your ribs. Count "one-two-three-one, one-two-three-two," and so on to ten.

Total time: 30 seconds.

Next comes the neck roll. Stand up straight. Without hunching your shoulders, tilt your head to one side and roll your head back and around until you're tilting it to the other side. Now go back. Do four rolls back, then four rolls to the front.

Total time: 30 seconds.

Now comes the lean and stretch. Again, stand straight, but this time place your feet a couple of feet apart. Leave one arm at your side and bring the other straight up over your head. Slowly lean in the direction opposite from the raised arm. Try to lean over without losing tension in your torso, yet still maintaining some flexibility in your body. Lean as far as you can, back off slightly, then lean again. Do this five times on one side, then five times on the other side. Repeat one more cycle of five on each side. If it feels better to keep your feet three feet apart, that's okay, too.

Total time: 30 seconds.

The next exercise I perform is a martial arts move that I don't recommend for beginners. It's no big deal, but it involves a certain amount of balance and you should probably not perform it without seeking an instructor. I went to a nearby junior college and took a self-defense class. The movement I was best at was the side kick, in which you turn sideways to your (imaginary) opponent, lift up your front leg, bending at the knee, while leaning over backward and sideways, away from your target. Then, you quickly straighten out your leg and bring it back to its bent position. By working with this movement for several months, I was able to combine it with a spin and a kick with the other leg.

Again, it is no great feat in and of itself, but it does require someone who is trained to judge your aptitude for balance to watch you and guide you.

Just for the record, the total time on this exercise is 45 seconds.

One alternative to this martial arts movement is a variation on the old running-in-place routine, but in this exercise you swing your feet out to the side with each step. It's kind of fun, because you build up a certain amount of pendulum action on both legs. Swing your arms across the front of your body while you move.

Total time: 45 seconds.

Although that was the first exercise where breath control might be a problem, you should practice breathing out during the point of maximum exertion in any exercise. The normal inclination is to suck air in, but this is wrong. Be certain to breathe out when exerting the most force, and your breathing inward will take care of itself.

Next are push-ups. I do fifteen of them on my knuckles while my hands are balled into fists, then I do five more in the conventional manner. Remember, you don't have to do all of these right at the start. Do one more each day. Do one more each week if you want to move that slowly. It doesn't matter how rapidly you take your exercise advancement as long as you do advance.

Total time on push-ups: one minute. (In case you're wondering about it, you do not touch the ground and rest in the middle of each push-up.)

The next exercise is performed while lying face down on the floor— exactly where you'll want to be after doing the push-ups. Stretch your arms out over your head and try to lift your hands/arms and feet/legs up off the ground as high as possible. I hold this position for 10 seconds, but I had to build up to that over time. Then I move my arms down to my sides and try to lift my hands/arms and feet/legs up from there while also lifting my head up and back. I do this for 10 seconds, too. Please don't try to do 10 seconds of these movements if you feel you're forcing yourself. I began doing these because of a back injury. I found that I did not experience any kinking up of my back if I performed these back stretches. Only after doing them for a couple of years did I realize that extending them for several seconds was also a good exercise.

Total time: 20 seconds for the actual work, but an additional minute to catch my breath.

Depending on how I feel about my tummy, I may or may not do this next one. Go back into the arms-up-in-front, legs-up-in-back pose and you can "walk" on your stomach for 10 seconds. Well, you can try.

Finally, I sometimes get into a sitting position, place the soles of my feet together, keep my back straight, and gently rock my bent knees down toward the floor.

Then, it's off to the shower. My exercise program lasts no more than six minutes a day, but the benefits are tremendous, and worth more to me than one two-hour workout a week.

14

Lose Weight Sitting Down

ALTHOUGH it is entirely possible that I am prejudiced in this matter, it is my contention that people who have desk jobs are quite special. And my respect and admiration, as well as the applicability of this chapter, extend to students, who spend so much of their time studying at desks; to homemakers who, although on their feet a lot, often sit down to do all those things that make theirs a desk job, too; and to anyone else whose day involves too much time spent seated, sedentary, or quiescent. (You know your own routine and circumstances best, so you should have little difficulty adapting my office-based examples to your particular situation.)

We use our brains rather than our brawn. That we frequently do not have any brawn to speak of is entirely beside the point. We get along in the world by putting our wits to work for us, unlike those big oafs who go barging through the world in the vain hope that might will somehow make right.

Weight and "heavyweight"

The only trouble with being desk-bound is the horrible tendency to get flabby in certain areas of the body. Since we do not throw our weight around (in the physical sense, I mean—some of the best Ego Diet users are "heavyweights" in their respective professions), we have to watch our weight. It's easy to let yourself go to the point of getting afflicted with the dreaded Desk Derriere or Front-office Fanny. (In case you have a fondness for these kinds of things, other choice epithets include Secretary Sag, Boardroom Bulk, Chair Cheeks, Professional Paunch, Push-button Paunch, and the ever popular Office Overgrowth.)

There are many opportunities for exercise while remaining in your office, but most people don't take advantage of them. Although it would be better to perform a regular series of exercises like those presented in Chapter 13 in tandem with the tricks outlined in this chapter, just doing these "gym-at-your-desk" exercises will be very beneficial.

Remember, you're not just battling the natural sloth that affects almost everyone in the atmosphere of the officeplace. You are also fighting your own bad habits. Then, too, you may have a hereditary problem to combat. Statistically, you have a 40 percent chance of being overweight if one of your parents was overweight. With both parents overweight the odds of your being too big double to 80 percent. (There is some disagreement over whether the effect of overweight parents is hereditary or environmental. For our purposes, the point is moot. All we care about is you and your well-being.)

The fun jobs

Everybody has some tasks that are more enjoyable than others. If you can save these up to do during what used to be your snack time, you'll be distracted from the food.

Think of these fun jobs as a reward for going through the day without sneaking a candy bar or doughnut.

The dirty jobs

I don't pretend to know why this works, but some people have told me they get through the day without all the between-meal nibbling by plunging into their most disagreeable task whenever the urge for a snack overtakes them.

Perhaps it's because they tense up over the dirty jobs and are thus less hungry. Or maybe it just takes more concentration of effort to tackle the bad jobs. Whatever the reason, the opposite reaction works for them.

You'll have to experiment and see which way makes the most sense (or makes the most distraction) for you.

Talk it up

You're sitting there mulling over a problem when suddenly you get the mouth-watering craves for a cup of coffee and a prepackaged snack cake. You know that's not good for you, but you can't get your mind back on the work at hand. That's not because the hunger is strong, it's because you need a mental break from the job.

Pick up the phone and call someone for a five-minute chat. It might be someone at work with whom you share a hobby. You can even call someone and talk about work, as long as it's a different task than the one with which you were just struggling. You need a change of pace, not a sweetcake in the face.

Dictation can sometimes take the place of a phone call. Get those letters you've been putting off out of the way. Put out some memos on items you've been meaning to discuss with people.

Get up

There's no rule that says you must stay at your desk all the time, is there? Go walk through the office in order to drop off something you'd normally send through the interoffice mail. You might meet a colleague along the way and get some other piece of business conducted. Or you might make a circuit of the place without meeting a soul. Either way, you got off your duff for a couple of minutes.

If you have a private place you can use, you can actually perform many of the exercises from Chapter 13 right in your office. Be careful not to do all of them at once or you'll work up a sweat. And, of course, unless you have a job on which you wear jeans (and the floors are kept clean), don't perform the "tummy walk" exercise.

While still seated

There are a number of good exercises you can do without even getting up from your desk. They work on the principle of isotonic contraction, which involves the use of a muscle or group of muscles without moving the body or changing the length of the muscle or muscles involved in the exercise.

Here are several of these exercises for you to try:

> ► *Chair pull*   Sit upright, spine straight and feet flat on the floor. Grip the bottom of your chair with your hands, making certain you have your hands placed on opposite sides of the middle of the seat of your chair. Slowly begin pulling upward with your arms. Do not use all your strength during this exercise (or in any of them where it seems you might tip or damage the furniture). The object isn't to go all out, just to provide tension for the muscles in your arms and shoulders. Find a point at which you can hold your arms tense for 30 seconds. Repeat two or three times a day or as needed.

▶ *Leg extenders*   Sit straight up in your chair and well balanced in the center. Place your hands as in the previous exercise, but instead of concentrating on your arms and shoulders, raise your legs, feet together, until they're parallel with the floor. Keep your back straight. Hold for 5 seconds. Repeat a couple of times a day.

▶ *Leg and arm resisters*   Sit upright in the middle of your chair, legs slightly apart and feet flat on the floor. Grip the bottom front part of your chair with your hands and slowly pull up with your arms while also pushing down with your legs. Hold for 10 seconds. Repeat two or three times a day.

▶ *Pretzel push*   If your chair has a leg that you can use, place your right foot on the left side of one leg. Now place your left foot on the right side of the same leg. Depending on the thickness of the chair, you can put your feet flat on the ground or brace yourself on the balls of your feet. Your legs will somewhat resemble a pretzel. Slowly apply pressure inward on the chair leg with both of your legs. Hold for 10 seconds. Now recross your legs so you adopt the same position but this time with your legs reversed. Hold for 10 seconds of pressure. Repeat twice a day.

Case history—a secretary

Sherry was eighteen years old when I first met her. She was excited about getting her first job as a secretary at a firm supplying speakers to college campuses, service clubs, and the like. Like a lot of people, she planned to take some evening college courses and work about three-quarter time during the day.

The first semester was great. She luxuriated in the relative freedom of attending classes only three nights a week, and in having some spending money of her own. The boutiques in the shopping malls also appreciated her ability to spend . . . given enough young ladies like Sherry, the owners of those shops could have retired early.

By buying her own clothes, cosmetics, and some meals, Sherry was also helping out at home. Her mother's income from a job in a travel agency was not high, her father had died some years before, and her younger brother was not old enough to get even a minimum wage part-time job. Sherry's extra income enabled her to do things that were previously only extravagances to be dreamed of, but were not to be considered seriously. Yet here she was, giddy as the breeze, bouncing from store to store, buying outfits to fit one new clothing fad after another, and loving every minute of it.

Suddenly it entered her mind that moving into her own apartment would be an exciting adventure. Her mother was dubious, but Sherry won her over.

"But Mom," she said, "it'll really help you. You won't have to worry about my meals or my laundry. . . ." Mom's eyes arched skyward a bit at this. The cliché about sons and daughters bringing dirty laundry home to mother is not a cliché for nothing. "And you won't have to lie awake waiting for me to come home from a date." Mom's eyes headed heavenward again. "But the best part is that you'll finally be able to turn my old bedroom into a sewing room." She struck paydirt. Mom liked that idea, and so Sherry got her own apartment amid much turmoil, penny-pinching, and tears of love.

The apartment wasn't much. Just two rooms. With an alcove for a dining area. Without much sunlight. In winter, it was freezing (and this was in California). In summer, it was an oven (it was still California). But Sherry loved it. It was a new way of life that was *adult*, and deliciously decadent.

Of course, with the added financial responsibilities of the lodging, and not wanting to cut way back on the collecting of fashion items for an ever-expanding wardrobe, she had to switch to a full-time job in order to bring in a fatter paycheck. The plans to complete college at night rapidly dissipated.

With her days now spent behind a desk and her nights free to go out to movies, Sherry entered into her most serious oral phase since early childhood. She ate her three regular meals, but they no longer comprised a balanced mixture of dairy, fruit and vegetable, grain, and protein items. Lunch and dinner often consisted of fastfood/junkfood. The introduction of fastfood breakfasts occurred at about this time, so there were days when Sherry gulped three junk meals in the space of ten hours.

Her eating didn't stop there, however. She was too smart to be satisfied with her relatively menial tasks at work, but she was pigeonholed as a secretary and therefore couldn't quickly make an upward move. Consequently, she was bored on her job. The boredom led to snacking. She began with sunflower seeds and raisins, which wouldn't have been bad if it had stopped right there.

When she found herself complaining about her weight while

clutching a Danish and a cup of sugared coffee, she freaked out and jumped at the first available weight-loss method she could find. Unfortunately, it was smoking. That partially satisfied her oral needs, but it also reinforced her dependence on oral "fixes" at regular intervals during the day.

Her nightly activities didn't help matters. Going to movies involved more sitting and more eating, what with the popcorn (buttered, of course) and other candy-counter goodies.

Sherry began going through a regular routine. Get up, get dressed, get depressed, go to work, get bored, eat, get mad, grab a junk food "meal," go out, snack, go home, get undressed, get depressed, go to bed. She was nervous and irritable all the time.

It was at this point in her life that she began to get The Idea. It had been with her for years, but The Idea was too private to talk about with other people. It was also unthinkable, both in the monetary sense and in the physical sense. The Idea, as she finally confided to me one night, was to totally remake herself in the image of a movie star.

"I want to be blonde," she said, "and beautiful."

"But you *are*—" I began.

"And have a big bust," she concluded abruptly.

"What?"

"I've always wanted to be bigger. You know, I even sent away for one of those 'bust developers' that you see advertised in the back of magazines."

"Not the magazines I read," I said.

"Oh. Yeah, right," she laughed. "Well, here, I'll show you," she said, leaning over to the coffee table, which was covered with fashion magazines, some envelopes, several invoices, a package of mascara, a box of tissue, a box of chocolate-covered nuts, and a hairbrush. Her purse had been sitting on it but had slid off for lack of a comfortable resting place.

"Look," she giggled. The ad said "Enlarge Your Bust!" in big block letters. The illustration that accompanied the ad looked like no woman I've ever seen. I said so.

"The bust on this babe," I told her, "would stop a train. You don't want to look like that, do you?"

She gave me a withering look, paused for a second, then got up and marched over to her closet. She took down a box from the top shelf, and opened it as she returned to the sofa.

"You know," she said, "this has always made me feel inadequate."

She held out the open box. Inside, nude, was a Barbie doll.

"You've got to be kidding," I said.

"Nope."

"This is insane," I said firmly. "No one wants to look like a phony plastic doll, even a big-chested one."

But it was no use. No amount of talk would dissuade her. She was going to dye her hair and "get a bust job" as she put it. She was saving her money for the operation, and had already talked to the plastic surgeon about it.

The only question seemed to be her weight and complexion. While she didn't actually come out and ask me for advice, I couldn't for the life of me figure out what other purpose I was invited there for, so I suggested we talk about her diet and exercise (or lack of exercise).

We discussed several of the points you've already read in this book, including the desk exercises in this chapter. She seemed particularly interested in these because she was smart enough to recognize that she was bored out of her skull at work. The opportunity to concentrate on something else was welcome, quite apart from the distraction from eating.

She asked about performing some of the morning exercises, especially the stretching ones, while at her desk. I told her that as long as her moving around in her chair wouldn't look funny to the others in her office, she could easily perform all but the floor exercises right there. It was at that point that I found out one more reason why she was so bored at work—she was the only one there for about 90 percent of the time. She had nothing to do for eight hours a day but type up travel plans and press releases and keep the books.

With the diet guidelines of The Ego Diet, plus the desk (and other) exercise plans, Sherry was able to lose the few excess pounds she had gained. This made her more confident, which in turn helped her relax a bit. I couldn't say whether or not The Ego Diet played a role, but she was promoted to field representative, which meant she got to travel with some of the speakers as well as enjoy much more responsibility on her job.

I'd like to say she realized how beautiful a woman she truly was and canceled her cosmetic surgery, but it just isn't so. The last time I saw her, she was the proud owner of a new set of breasts. Her hair was that brittle lemon-yellow from too much bleaching, but her waist was twenty-three inches and her complexion was clear and bright. But there was something odd about her, something oddly out of place. Then it came back to me. She looked like a Barbie doll.

Case history—an executive

Nancy was a rebel. She ran away from home when she was seventeen, hitched rides across this country and much of Canada, joined an informal motorcycle gang (and has the tattoo to prove it), and faked her way into one of this country's larger corporations at the junior executive level.

After spending a rather wild eighteen months living life on the road, Nancy became disgusted with herself and her current friends. As she put it, "I was bugged by always having to pretend to less knowledge than I had, just to get along without starting arguments. Some of those people are fundamentally fine but what they know about psychology and middle-class motivations wouldn't fill a gnat's navel."

She was in the middle of one of their more and more frequent arguments when an offhand remark from one of the bikers sparked her into action. "I don't think he really knew what he was saying," she relates, "but he in essence challenged me to prove some of the points I had been making about the way American business works. I guess he figured none of us would ever know what the inside of a boardroom looked like, so his challenge couldn't be met. That's when I took off for Harvard."

Nancy applied to the Harvard Business School and went on to receive her M.B.A., a treasured document to would-be corporate executives. She moved to the West Coast, went on job interviews, and as a lark filled out one application form with erroneous information. She altered part of her name, changed her college, put down the address of a friend, and outright faked her typing and dictation skills. She got into the interview and instead of acting reserved and eager as she had on her other interviews, she was just herself: smart, but also a smark aleck. She was funny, flippant, aggressive, and annoying. And they hired her to join the typing pool. Perhaps the personnel director saw her ultimate worth to the company. Perhaps he just thought it was a wonderful joke to hire her. We will never know. All we do know is that within six months she had every secretary loathing her and every executive to whom she was assigned loving her work. She corrected their mistakes, contributed suggestions that made them look good, and generally did about 120 percent of her job.

She was given a promotion to junior assistant coordinator of something or other. "It was just a bogus title," she states, but she figured out a way to turn that to her advantage. "Nobody had ever heard of the position I held, and nobody had ever bothered to define the parameters of the job, so I just . . . Took Over." She gets a gleam in her eye when she tells this story. "I asked for information from every middle-level manager in the company. I read it all, on the bus, in the bathroom, at lunch, in bed. Pretty soon, I knew how the company worked. Who was good at what they did, and who was lousy. Who was going to succeed on certain projects, and who was going to fail. Most important, I knew *why*.

"So I began drafting memos to people in the company. A suggestion here, a recommendation there. A summary report. A preliminary finding. A prediction. People began to notice my stuff. Of course, some of it made them mad, but I just used that as the basis of a psychological profile report. One man came storming into my office with one of my reports crumpled in his fist, yelling his head off. I just took out my mini tape player, switched it on, laid it on the desk, and began taking notes on a big clipboard. He got real silent, real fast. I just said 'Out!' and he left. I never saw him again."

Then she really struck gold. "I saw a memo that the Vice-Chairman of the company was considering an invitation to speak at an upcoming convention. That week, I wrote the best damn speech he ever saw. I sent it to his office with a note about how I had taken his advice about writing him a few words for use at some later date. I alluded to a phone conversation we had a couple of months ago. He loved the speech. I got to move up again."

That was five years ago. In the meantime, Nancy has gone through three apartments and two condominiums on her way to being a vice-president in her company. The only problem she encountered along the way was an eating problem that stemmed from her insecurity over being the youngest corporate executive at her firm, and one of very few females to boot.

She began soothing herself with snacks, calming herself down with minimeals between meals. Although she was driven to do more than anyone else at work, she was able to take in more food than she needed by eating something every chance she got.

"I was a pig," she puts it bluntly. "I ate everything that even looked like it belonged on a plate. It's a good thing nobody brought any of that plastic joke food because I probably would have gobbled that down, too."

Nancy and I talked for several hours over the course of a couple of weeks. She resisted every Ego Diet method I suggested. Finally, in desperation, I brought up the desk exercises. From her description of her work habits, I assumed that she was hopping around the building all day long, but that was far from the case. It turned out that she was desk-bound far more often than not. She may have been bombarding everyone with directives, summaries, and reports, but she did it from behind her desk.

She pounced on the exercises with maniacal glee. "That's what I need!" she exclaimed. She made me demonstrate every one on the spot, then she tried them all with a seriousness every teacher would love to see in every pupil.

Nancy used the desk exercises every day. Her weight went back down to her ideal level and she didn't rely so much on eating for a security blanket. "Now," she states, "whenever I feel upset or unsure of myself, I grab my chair with one of your exercises. It takes my mind off the problem or it lets me get out some anger by using my muscles."

Case history—the perpetual student

Barbara was a thin girl in high school. Almost too thin. She certainly was too thin in one area that she thought was important for attracting boys. Unlike Sherry, who didn't have anything to worry about in this area, Barbara was indeed flat-chested. She entered college in search of a man, was unsuccessful, dropped out, went to work, saved up enough money for cosmetic surgery, and went out to rebuild herself. A new nose. New breasts. And a new outlook on food. She thought she would gain a more alluring body if she could only add a few pounds to her too-slim hips. She went back to college with her new face and body and about four pounds of high-protein powder for "weight shakes" that she'd whip up in a blender.

Thirty-eight pounds later, she realized she had gone too far. An odd thing had happened while she was attracting the boys: she began to get interested in the classes she was taking. A very bright person, Barbara had been able to get A's and B's without doing much studying. All of her energy went toward getting dates. Now that the dates were readily available, she found that the history, geology, biology, English, and physics she had been ignoring were pretty fascinating.

Of course, the attention she got from the guys in her classes dropped off as she added pounds, and she wanted to stop gaining weight. "It's not so much because of the guys," she said. "Oh I like to be popular, and I want to go out with one certain guy, but I also want to continue in school and get my bachelor's, then go on for a master's. I want to go into research. I like studying, and that way I can continue. But I'm afraid that this is going to leave me like a blimp because I never get any exercise."

Out came the notes for this chapter. Barbara began doing exercises at her school desk. She also discovered that she had been eating in class without even thinking about it. "I was surprised to find I had four candy bars in my purse. The girl I sit next to in history told me I ate one or two every day she saw me."

That was something Barbara stopped when she started doing her desk exercises. She used the hunger as a signal to perform one of the exercises. Her weight went back down. She went out on the dates she wanted. The last I heard of her, she was working on a research project for a Canadian television company and was about to get married . . . to someone she had helped lose weight with the desk exercises.

15

Laughter Helps

THERE are twenty-two bones in your head. Only one moves—the lower jaw—and it's part of your face. Of the twenty-one other bones that form your head, fourteen are part of your face. As you can see by studying yourself with two mirrors placed at a 45-degree angle to one another, your face comprises a relatively small percentage of your head, yet all but a third of the head's bones go into the structure and design of your face.

There are three groups of muscles on your head. One is the group of muscles you hardly use: the muscles of your scalp. It is unusual to find people who can wiggle their ears or scalp voluntarily, on command; only animals have retained the ability to make regular use of these muscles. The other two groups of muscles on your head—those dealing with the eyes and eyelids, and those around your lips—are facial muscles.

Why is the face so important that it warrants this disproportionate attention? Some people believe it is because your face mirrors the way you feel, and the multitude of expressions available to you represents the multitude of emotional states in which you can find yourself. Others believe that it is exactly the reverse, that you first act out the visualization of the emotion which follows. While neither theory has yet been proved (and the truth could possibly lie somewhere in between), it may be that the latter theory, despite sounding a bit less likely, may be closer to reality. The fact is that your emotions are somewhat related to what your face is showing; of course, it is also true that your face shows a lot of what you feel (you see why neither theory can be proved). Everyone agrees that, in certain instances, you do react emotionally in accordance with your facial commands.

If you are asked "How are you?" your response may actually affect the way you feel. The person who answers with a smile and a pleasant "Fine!" and a hearty "How's yourself?" is much more likely to truly feel better than that same person would if the answer was a morose "Oh, okay, I guess . . ."

That your face may be considered the "mirror of the mind" is not so farfetched. (The entire quotation is "The face is the mirror of the mind, and eyes without speaking confess the secrets of the heart." It is from St. Jerome.) You may remember the times you misjudged a person from his or her appearance, but this is because it is out of the ordinary for people to be different from the way they look. While it is true that you cannot tell the difference between a convict and a chaplain when both are dressed alike, you can tell the difference based on the way they act when they don't think you're watching them. And by "the way they act," I mean the way their faces look.

You can always tell the truly fine actors in films and plays because they're the ones who show what their characters are thinking and feeling whenever they *aren't* talking. To a certain extent, this is something to watch for in real life. When people don't think they are the center of attention, they look different. They relax a bit and become closer to their true selves. Glance at individuals who are trying to convince you of something that seems dubious or is going to cost you money. Take a good sharp look at them when they stop to let you talk. Try to put the conversation on hold for some reason, like having to make an important phone call. Just say it won't take a minute, pick up the phone and pretend to buzz someone about a lunch appointment or whatever. Watch how they look, especially if you have been going along with them up to this point. You may find that there is a distasteful "I've just hooked another sucker" look on such a person's face.

Your inner emotions tend to come out on your face. In adolescence, this is seen in your facial reaction to your inner turmoil: pimples. This time of life is so full of ups and downs—everything is *crucial*, everything is almost a matter of life and death—that they become evident, even on the faces of those who are blessed with pure skin. In adulthood, there are more social pressures to hide your emotions. You're not supposed to show that you don't like someone at work (especially if it's the boss). You're not able to truthfully answer questions like "Do you like my new hairstyle?" when asked of you by a thirty-nine-year-old overweight housewife who has just gone punk. Yet your emotions still present themselves to the astute observer in a myriad of subtle ways. The slight tic around the eyes. The faint "glazing over" of the eyes as your thoughts turn inward. The sideward glance. The almost imperceptible tightening of the lips or the area around the mouth. The signs are there despite our trying valiantly to conceal them.

It has long been a staple of Sunday School wisdom that "it takes more effort to frown than to smile because frowning uses more muscles." This is said, apparently, in the hope that more people will smile because they enjoy using fewer muscles. It's the school of thought that states that people will do anything if they think they're missing some work. I'm positive this doesn't have any validity or everyone would be wandering around smiling and just tickled pink at saving all that effort of frowning. One glance out any window will tell you that isn't happening.

It isn't happening because we all have frowning forced into us as the only right and true way to go through life. We're taught very early in life that laughter isn't "good." We must not laugh in school (which means we're taught right away that learning isn't fun—an absolutely wrongheaded way to raise people). We must not laugh in church (which means we're taught that faith isn't supposed to be uplifting, despite what we *say* religion is supposed to be about). We mustn't laugh in so very many Important Places or on so very many Important Occasions that it's no wonder that, as adults, we frown a lot.

We frown to indicate we're thinking. And this means that we eventually come to the point where we actually do frown when we're thinking. We also frown to indicate sadness, irritation, disapproval, skepticism, sarcasm, anger, and some forms of fear.

From the beginning, we close ourselves off to a healthy, youth-giving, life-giving release of natural emotion: the joy of laughter. Smiling and laughing can make you feel better mentally and improve your body physically. Some terminally ill patients have reversed their decline and made substantial progress toward recovery after embarking on a "joyful happiness search," as one of them put it. We all should take a journey of rediscovery of the simple pleasures of life and the peace that comes from being able to laugh at the vagaries of life.

Certainly there will be sadness in your life. You will experience the same heartbreaks and losses that millions of others have faced in the past and millions will face in the future. You will get depressed from time to time. And angry. But if you can work out the anger and frustration instead of bottling it up inside, you have a better chance to enjoy your life.

If you can change all the "teaching" you have received about being serious, if you can get yourself to the point of accepting laughter into your life, you'll be on the road to extending your life and feeling younger. You may not alter your chronological age, but you can vastly improve your psychological age. When you feel younger, you act younger. These two things together are a potent way to make you a healthier person.

You might be able to get yourself to laugh at the uproarious predicaments in which we continually find ourselves. "Life, she is a human comedy," as an immigrant friend of mine was fond of putting it. By laughing at the absurdities of this world, you might be able to get yourself to the point of laughing about the toughest subject of all: yourself.

Good exercise

True, fewer muscles are taxed by smiling, but a big grin or a laugh uses lots of facial muscles and tummy muscles. The muscles that criss-cross your torso at stomach level are utilized during laughter. The phrase, "I laughed until my sides hurt" is common precisely because laughing exercises muscles you use infrequently.

So laugh it up, folks. Have a *good* time tonight, partners. If you cringe at some of what follows, it may be because it strikes a little too close to home. If so, try to keep it in mind the next time you get hungry. Use your reaction—which may be simple embarrassment—to good advantage by recalling it when tempted to overeat or when tempted to eat the wrong foods.

If you just find these stories amusing, then that's fine, too. Hope you use lots of muscles with every chuckle.

Spreading out the holiday treats
(or spreading out from them)

There is a funky, hand-drawn, oversize greeting card that is pasted to the wall of the kitchen in the ad agency where I work. It came to us from a client as part of a thank-you gift for our efforts on behalf of their four-day ski show. Being a once-a-year event, it is not the size of account that we would normally accept, but they are nice people who often let us do whatever we want in the creation of their advertising, so it's too much fun to pass up.

We handle their show every year, so there is a strange kind of conti-nuity to our relationship. As the years go by, our outside interests change. When we were younger, we thought nothing of doing the radio commercials at night, with a pizza and beer brought into the studio. Now that we all have noticed our bellies don't like that kind of treatment (both in the sense of digestion and in added inches), we take a much different approach to the timing of our recording sessions.

Still, we all enjoy food, especially those special treats that are available around Christmas time. We were talking about the coming holiday season (the ski show is held in September or October), and how we wished we could spread out the sugary goodies over several months rather than having them crammed into a brief six-week period. Knowing this, they sent us a tray of dessert items along with the drawing. The food disappeared almost instantly, but the drawing remains up to this day. It shows a plump girl with the caption "Remember, you can always suck in your stomach, but you can't suck in your thighs."

What kind of food am I?

A game that went around among all my friends a while ago—like the trivia game seemed to grab everybody—involved a simple question. If you had to describe yourself as a piece of food, what kind of food would you be?

I said I was an apple, although several others disagreed and suggested many different varieties of nuts.

The most interesting response and reaction occurred with a slightly overweight friend named Ned. He described himself as being "a Sara Lee dessert product." We naturally asked which Sara Lee product in particular. "All of 'em," he said.

One of the other people thought about that for a while, then commented, "Well, I guess that makes sense. Those things are delicious, but not very good for you."

"Oh, thanks," replied Ned.

But the comment had a certain validity. Being around Ned was a disaster for people trying to control their diet.

The session broke up with someone singing "what kind of food am I?" to the tune of "What Kind of Fool Am I?"

Quickies

These put-downs, bits of sarcasm, and one-liners are a bit mean, and they were designed to ridicule someone. As such, they are not the kind of humor I usually favor. Yet, for some reason, these struck me funny when I heard them the first time. Perhaps it had to do with the timing of the person delivering them, or the situation in which they were used.

I know that they didn't hurt quite so much because they weren't directed at me, even though I was overweight when most of them first surfaced. Some of them would float into my mind as I contemplated eating something, and they helped me smile at my own foibles and weaknesses (and they helped me decide to avoid some bad foods, too).

> Delivered as an offhand remark in a deadpan manner: "Say, either you're gaining a little weight or you're working up to audition for the Pillsbury Doughboy." (Variation on this involves the Michelin Tire symbol and, of course, Santa Claus.)

> Shopclerk, bored with the fussiness of an overweight woman customer: "Well, whatever you do, don't wear a red dress or you'll have the whole fire department trying to put you out."

> Helpful hint from one spouse to another: "I sure wouldn't recommend wearing gray on an ocean voyage . . ." (Pause for the other person to ask, "Why?") "Because the Navy pilots will try to land planes on you."

> Liz Taylor's bumper sticker: "Honk if you have food."

The bum's rush

Among the higher class of the down-and-outers there exists a sub-culture complete with rules, etiquette, slanguage, signs and symbols, and folklore. One piece of the bum's folklore has it that fatter ladies are more likely to be a soft touch for free meals than most other people.

One up-and-coming young tramp, hearing this, asked for some examples. The others around the campfire told him that overweight women "of a certain age" were by nature good-hearted fools willing to give unhesitatingly and without reserve.

Feeling buoyant with this new and precious information, our young tramp set out into town to find himself a meal ticket. Spying a well-endowed matron outside a store, he went into his best act.

"Madame, may I have a moment of your time? I'm getting desperate. You see, I haven't touched any food at all for three whole days. Think of it, seventy-two solid hours without eating."

"Oh my," exclaimed the woman, "I admire your will power."

Overlooking something

When his wife came to ask for more money "for groceries," Sam the accountant totaled up in his mind the amounts of money that were going out and balanced them against the minor sums that were coming in. He didn't like the bottom line.

Although normally a mild-mannered man, Sam was determined to have his wife get more responsible in her food-buying habits. He gently and wisely suggested that Esther be more frugal.

"Frugal, schmugal," she replied, "we need more food in this house."

Sam became exasperated. "Just where on earth is all the grocery money going?" he demanded.

"Just turn sideways and look in the mirror," she demanded back. "For heaven's sake, Sam, coming from a man who can't see his shoes when he's standing up, you sure are overlooking where all our food is going."

Sassy machinery

The talk of the town was the new "talking scale" down at the barber shop. "It speaks your weight!" cried the banner across the front of the mechanical marvel.

One after another, the townspeople stepped up on its gleaming, machine-tooled weight plate. And the crowd of idle shopkeepers, retirees, hangers-on, and genuine barber shop customers would press closer in anticipation of the wisecrack commentary spewed forth for the price of a nickel. For this set of scales not only converted your weight into computer synthesized speech, it also made some sort of observation about the weight of the people getting on.

The good folks getting their kicks from the talking scale had to find out two things. First, they wanted to know if the machine would repeat a message. As nickel after nickel disappeared into the shiny coin-deposit slot, the anticipation and awe increased. The machine seemed to have a response for everyone. True, it didn't seem to know the sex of the weighee, and it couldn't tell if the people with the lower weights were children or just small adults. Yet most of the comments were on target. When Willie the barber got on, the machine said, "You weigh one hundred eighty-two pounds. I hope you're tall enough for that weight." Everybody laughed at that because Willie was almost offered a basketball scholarship a few years back when he was barely graduating from high school. When Mama Shirley got up on it, the strange, stilted mechanical voice told her (and the crowd of eager faces squeezing ever closer), "Your weight is one hundred twenty-one pounds . . . with your clothes on this time." That really broke up the place. Everyone knew that Mama Shirley was once caught in a raid of the town's service club "smoker" when they had hired her to jump out of a cake.

After a while, the jokes didn't seem to be as funny. Maybe they were getting tired of hearing the odd, pinched, metallic voice. Or maybe it was just too much of a good thing. The murmur of voices began discussing the second item on the agenda: Could the machine be broken? A call was put in for Wilson, the biggest man in the county.

Wilson jiggled when he walked. People got off the sidewalk when Wilson came rolling and bouncing slowly down the avenue. When there was thunder, folks would smile and say that Wilson was trying to play jump rope or hopscotch.

So when Wilson waddled up onto the scale, there was more than the usual hush in the packed room. Slowly, deliberately, Wilson placed a nickel in the slot, dropped it, and . . . nothing happened. Then, out of the strained silence, the machine said calmly, "One at a time, please."

Ready-maid diet

The wealthy women who gathered for tea once a week had several surefire topics of conversation. They talked about each other's husbands, about their own weight, their new clothes, and what they termed "the servant problem." When two of these topics could be combined, it was a banner day.

This particular day didn't look like it was going to be out of the ordinary. One member of the regular group was missing, but that was to be expected because everyone thought she was out of town as she had been the previous week. So it was a surprise when she showed up. And a double surprise when she showed up looking slimmer than usual.

The other ladies gathered around, firing questions at her left and right: "Did you go to a fat farm?" "Are you taking pills?" "Is a doctor supervising your diet?" "What is your diet, anyway?"

They were caught up short when they heard the truth. "It's none of those things," she said with a sigh. "It's just that I'm having so much trouble with my new maid that I can't eat for worry."

After making the appropriate sounds of sympathy, they asked why she didn't just fire the maid?

"Oh I can't do that," she cried, "not until she worries me down another twelve pounds."

The inside story

When the overweight woman got on the broken scale, the needle swung around to forty-five pounds and stopped cold. A drunk wandering past took in the sight of this large woman on the scale, squinted at the indicator, then muttered in amazement, "She's hollow."

Good advice

If you're overweight, carefully regulate your intake of food, but cut back. In fact, you might look at it this way: Don't eat, fast.

If you're at your ideal weight, look at it this way: Don't eat fast.

Are fat people jolly?

That's the cliché. Jolly Saint Nick, and countless others. But is it true in real life? Many times, overweight people are trying to live up to the cliché. They feel they're more acceptable to others if they laugh it up.

This is forced laughter, and it does not help as much as the genuine article. Try to find books, plays, films, and television shows that make you hold your sides with laughter. Roll your head back and let the laughter come rolling out until the tears cloud your eyes.

Laughter is good medicine.

16

A Few Words About Cancer

WHEN I was growing up, one of the delightful aspects of our family having a big dinner of turkey was the cleaning of the wishbone and hanging it up above the stove to dry. After a few days, my mother would deem it ready and the two of us would grab one end each, pause to make a wish, and pull. Whoever ended up with the top joint still connected to the "handle" was the winner, and the silent wish would come true. When we first began playing this game, we would each win about the same number of times in each year. Since my wishes were almost always for material things, perhaps this was just as well, for I had plenty of toys, and, being an only child, I received quite a bit of attention.

As I grew a little older, I began seeing the results of suffering in the world. One word that seemed to affect more people we knew or were related to was cancer. I asked about cancer and read about it in the school library. Thus I learned that cancer, in any form, is an abnormal growth of cells in the body. As the cancer cells multiply, they take over from your own healthy tissue. There were lots of "cures" and yet no cure, because we didn't know why some cancers could be stopped and others kept growing.

After learning about cancer, I changed my silent wish every time my mother and I grabbed a wishbone. I asked for a cure for cancer. I began winning most of the wishbone tug o' wars. That was fun, but unfortunately my wishes have not yet come true.

What we "know" about cancer

During the past ten or fifteen years, much has been written about cancer. Many so-called facts about cancer have been printed in many different types of publications, and much has been said on television and radio talk shows. So much of this information has been simply a rehash of earlier information that we've all come to "know" certain things about cancer.

If you ask most people about the causes of cancer, they may tell you a few specifics, but they will probably tell you that most cancer is caused by either smoking or synthetic substances. The figure that is often used these days is 90 percent of all cancer is caused by industrial chemicals. Some people also state that we are in the midst of an epidemic of industrially caused cancer.

Why do people believe these things to be true? Because they've read about it in their newspapers and heard about it on TV. But in a book by Edith Efron, all these facts are disputed. She points out that evidence exists that our Earth is filled with natural carcinogens (cancer-causing agents), that industrially caused cancer accounts for under 30 percent of all cancers, and that the incidence of cancer is no higher as a percentage of the population than it was years ago (although more cancer is detected prior to patients becoming terminal).

In short, we don't even know what we don't know about cancer.

Cancer and healthy bodies

There are direct carcinogens which may do damage to your body right away. Certain cancer viruses fall into this category. We don't yet know who is most susceptible to these agents, but we do know a little about who is susceptible to indirect carcinogens, such as chemicals in foods. One reason for this is the path the indirect carcinogens must follow in order to cause cancer to begin growing in your body. They must pass the normal defenses against disease. The membranes, enzymes, and natural antibodies all put up some resistance. Such factors as your age, general health, diet, and mental condition all have some effect. If you're in a weakened state, you're more likely to suffer cancer, just as is the case with other, more conventional diseases.

The healthier you are, the lower your odds of getting cancer. The better your diet, the healthier you are. Therefore, the better your diet, the less chance you have of getting cancer.

Mental condition

I have been close to two victims of cancer. From this admittedly very small sample, I have drawn some conclusions about potential cancer victims, because of the similarities in their cases. Nothing I have read on the subject refutes my findings, but I must point out that a great deal of study remains to be done in this area, and that my observations are hardly scientific evidence. Still, I firmly believe the mental "set" of these two people contributed to their contracting cancer.

Dan was my boss at a small company he owned back in the 1960s. His whole life was practically the antithesis of The Ego Diet. He treated food as something to be gobbled up at any time of the day or night. He paid no attention to what kind of food it was as long as it "tasted good," which meant, more often than not, fried and greasy food or food with a high sugar content. There was never the slightest consideration given to the speed of consumption or elegance of setting.

His self-image was as perverted as his attitude toward food. The man went through his adult life suspecting the worst of everybody he met. While he expected consideration and respect from others (and sulked when it was not forthcoming), he never gave one second's thought for the feelings of others.

Fortunately for me, he was also lazy, so as soon as I demonstrated an ability to run his small business, he spent less and less time at the office. This greatly improved the working conditions, as you can imagine. He did pop in unannounced from time to time, snatching up papers from people's desks in order to see what was going on at that moment. I once asked him why he bothered to do that, because it was annoying and it was causing a turnover in secretaries. He looked a bit sheepish and muttered something about "checking up on people because they're not honest."

I found out later that he constantly speculated at home about how people he knew weren't being honest in their personal relationships with him. His wife told me he would wonder out loud whether people really liked him or if they were merely pretending to like him. Which was odd, because people would have been able to like him better if he wasn't the sort of bloke who was suspicious about whether people liked him or not. And, since he didn't trust us, his employees, enough to leave our work in place on our desks, he was hardly in a position to complain about others not being honest with him.

At this point, you might be thinking that it was no great loss when this man died of cancer a few years later. Certainly there was not a great deal of grieving at his passing. Yet, it was still sad. Here was a man who spent his adult life looking over his shoulder at imaginary ghosts. He wasn't really alive, in my opinion.

Please understand that his distasteful habits are not the point—his not allowing himself to realize the pleasures of life and his diabolical approach to food were factors that contributed to the diseased condition of his body. I am not suggesting that the "bad" people in the world are more likely to get cancer, as you'll see in the next few paragraphs.

What I am suggesting is that the wrong attitude toward life and the wrong approach to the fuel of life will increase your chances of getting cancer.

I know a beautiful and good person who has cancer at this moment. She has had seven operations for cancer in the past ten years. Her personal habits bear as much resemblance to Dan's as an iceberg to a pile of lint. Yet she still shares something with Dan, something I believe was a factor in her getting cancer, albeit at a much later stage in life (she is now in her seventies).

Actually, she shares two things with Dan, the first being a less than perfect diet. She is in no way as guilty of eating bad foods, but she did not group foods properly. Her meals would often be high in protein and vegetables but exclude grain, dairy products, and fruits. And this might continue for several main meals in a row. She also had very little variety in her preparation and presentation of food. There just was the one way for her to do it, and she was not interested in one of the true delights of cooking: the gentle art of experimentation with recipes.

More important, hers was a rather rigid view of life. She was raised by a very religious family that allowed for no gray areas in the judgment of human behavior. What's right is right and what's wrong is wrong was their motto. While that sort of knee-jerk reaction may have been helpful back on the prairie when we were building this nation from the soil up, it does not fit in contemporary society with its shifting standards of behavior and its generally amoral stance regarding personal behavior that doesn't harm anyone else.

Her own rigidity was inhibiting, both to herself and to those around her. She is a bright, witty, and charming woman, yet her timid approach to anything new is almost sad to see. Her view of life was an old one even before she was old—she rejected anything that represented change and accepted everything that was fmiliar.

Like Dan, she was not fully alive for much of her adult life. And this is something that may greatly affect the body's ability to deal with the abnormal cell growth known as cancer.

Once, when she was over at our house, my wife put a couple of chairs out on the balcony so several of us could sit and watch over the valley. We all bounded in and out of our chairs, dashing on and off the balcony to talk, get something to drink, change a cassette on the stereo, and so forth. Suddenly I became aware that only one person was still sitting on the balcony. She had a pleasant, peaceful expression on her face as she sat and watched the world go by. A bird flew across our yard and landed in a treetop on a direct line with the top of the balcony. She happily watched it until it flew off into the distance and disappeared. Eventually the spell was broken and she rejoined us inside the house. The same inhibitions again surfaced. But for those few moments, this lovely woman seemed more alive to me than in several years of knowing her. I cannot help but think that if she could have accepted more of life with that same sense of wonder and awe she would not have contracted cancer. Perhaps with the strong mental outlook, she would have had a stronger immune system to fight off the malignancy.

I hope that someday soon my wishbone wishes come true.

Cancer and vitamins

Can the right vitamins help prevent cancer? Some doctors believe so. Many studies have shown that people whose diet includes foods rich in vitamins C and E have less cancer overall and much less cancer of the digestive tract. Some physicians and scientists believe that the two vitamins work in combination to protect your healthy body cells from the ravaging effects of cancer cells.

The walls of the cells in your body are living membranes with connections to every other cell structure. They are also interfacing with the cell walls of other cells all around them. Each cell is a signal and control center, and many cells together combine to perform similar signal and control functions in your body. Toxic substances, which enter your body through foods, affect your cells. Usually, the cells win in the battle against the toxic by-products of fats, oils, grease, and chemicals from the food you eat. But if they don't win, metabolism in the cell produces something called a free radical, which can damage your cells so much that a cancer cell emerges.

Vitamins C and E apparently help shield cells from this devastating effect. As you'll see in the chapter on vitamins, it is better to get them into your body through eating vitamin-rich foods rather than by taking vitamin supplements. In general, whole grains, fresh fruits, and fresh vegetables are the best sources of C and E.

An anticancer diet

The American Cancer Society has called for the establishment of an anticancer diet. Most of their recommendations for such a diet have been incorporated into this book. In general, they make several points about the things you put into your body:

> ► Eat less fat, oil, and smoked foods.
> ► Eat more fiber and vegetables.
> ► Avoid smoking.
> ► Reduce consumption of alcohol.

A number of eating practices and specific foods are discussed in the next few pages. While some are proven carcinogens and others are proven cancer-inhibitors, there are some foods on the list about which science only has suspicions. In the cases where there is some doubt, I've mentioned that the food is only suspected of causing cancer or helping to cause cancer. Again, I want to stress that you do not have to completely avoid these foods, just be aware of your intake of them and do not overdo it.

Alcohol
Don't drink.

According to the International Agency for Research on Cancer, a group that is part of the World Health Organization, even an average drinker is increasing the odds of getting cancer of the mouth, larynx, pharynx, and esophagus. It is the ethanol that is the cause. Ethanol is a substance present in ethyl alcohol.

Barbiturates
There is some suspicion that barbiturates like phenobarbital and barbital tend to promote the cause of cancerous tumors.

Barbiturates are found in tranquilizers and sleeping pills.

Cigarettes and smoking
Don't smoke.

In particular, don't smoke cigarettes.

Cigarette smoking (whether by the individual or by others in the area who are forced to breathe the same smoke-filled air) has been implicated in a majority of cases of oral cancers of all types, lung cancer, emphysema, and cancers of the larynx, pharynx, and bladder.

Cosmetics
More than one hundred ingredients in various cosmetics are suspected of promoting cancer and birth defects. Fortunately, the Food and Drug Administration is investigating cosmetics and their means of

manufacture, and some products are being altered or removed from the market. Still, they cannot move fast enough in all cases at once, so moderation is best in this area.

Lotions, skin creams, shampoos, and other facial cosmetics are among those products being tested, although the worst products appear to be hair colorings and hair dyes.

Hair dye

The synthetic dyes used in the most popular hair-coloring preparations are now suspected to contain cancer-causing agents. If you feel you must alter your hair color, it is best to avoid the methods that touch your scalp. Streaking or frosting your hair does not involve the scalp. Some hair coloring products have had the suspected ingredients removed. If you can find a listing of ingredients on the product you wish to use, these are the dyes to avoid: 2-nitro-p-phenylenediamine, 4-nitro-o-phenylenediamine, C1 acid black, azo dye with 4-amino-2-nitrophenol, 4-methoxy-m-phenylenediamine, 4-MMPD, 2, 4-toluene diamine, 4-amino-2-nitrophenol, 2-nitrophenylenediamine, direct black 38, direct blue 6, and 2, 4-diaminoanisole.

Emotion

Psychological studies of cancer patients reveal some similarities among many of them. Their relationships with their parents were usually more cool and aloof than average. They are more likely to be people who keep their feelings bottled up inside rather than finding ways to let off steam (both anger and affection are "steam" in this case). The more repressed the person in terms of sex, the more likely the incidence of cancer. In general, those people who are not afraid to display their love or their anger have a better chance of fighting against cancer. Patients who were able to become angry at their illness did better than those who were pliant or resigned to their fate. As Dylan Thomas said in his poem to his father, "Do not go gentle into that good night, . . . Rage, rage, against the dying of the light."

Diet

As previously mentioned, your diet may be able to help your body ward off cancer. Among the foods that have been associated with cancer are: foods pickled in salt or preserved in salt; beef; fat; and foods that are exceedingly spicy.

Certain dietary deficiencies, such as a lack of vitamins, also apparently foster cancer. Lack of vitamin A, magnesium, and iodine may contribute to cancer.

On the other hand, vitamins C and E seem to help prevent cancer, as do the chemicals found naturally in plants such as broccoli, brussels sprouts, turnips, and cauliflower. (There is some irony in the fact that plants from the mustard family may help prevent cancer, while mustard may help cause it.)

Food flavorings—a cause of cancer?

The flavoring agents in such harsh foods as mustard, horseradish, and pepper have been shown to cause cancer. This does not mean you should instantly stop using pepper on your eggs. The amount of harsh food flavoring doesn't add up to a tablespoon a day for the average American. But if you're tempted to add more and more of this kind of food to your diet, don't. It could be dangerous.

The normal amounts of these foods will start an attack on your cell walls. They actually smash holes in the cellular lining, thus setting you up for the growth of cancer. Your body's defense mechanism against this form of attack is the natural shedding of the lining of your digestive system on a daily basis. You can easily see that too much of this sort of thing and your body just cannot cope.

Other types of flavoring to watch for include the charred sections of overly cooked meat, fish, toast, and bread crust. If you like to sear your meat, just avoid eating the part that looks like charcoal. Carmelized sugar is also to be taken only in moderation.

Cancer and fat

The average person in America now consumes fats and oils to the tune of 40 percent of the total calorie intake each day. Fats and oils do make foods taste smoother, creamier, moister, and richer. Unfortunately, they also seem to cause cancer.

In order for your body to digest fat, something called bile acids are formed. It is suspected that bile acids actually cause the cancer, but it is fat that's the trigger.

Cancer of the breast and of the bowel have been linked to diets with high fat and oil intake. Protests from the Meat Marketing Board notwithstanding, it would be better for you if you cut down on the amount of hot dogs, hamburgers, sausages, and cold cuts you eat, for all of these contain very high percentages of fat.

There are other prices we pay for having the highest fat intake of any nation in civilized history. Among them are obese bodies, heart disease, and more bowel problems. However, the risk of having cancer get a hold on your body—even if it is twenty years from now—seems to outweigh these concerns, strong though they may be.

Fiber

Over the last century, the average American diet has had an 80 percent drop in the amount of fiber eaten. We have literally learned not to eat foods with fiber. Yet there is now evidence that a high-fiber diet can help prevent cancer by helping remove foreign substances from the intestine.

Almost all fiber foods are carbohydrates, but fiber is a type of carbohydrate that humans cannot digest. The best fibers are insoluble—they do not dissolve in water. When you eat fiber, it creates bulk in your digestive tract. This bulk speeds your body's elimination process, thus helping to cleanse your system more rapidly. It also makes elimination easier (with the helpful side effect of lessening the occurrence of hemorrhoids).

You might think of the soluble fibers as passing through your system like a sponge, soaking up excess water and many impurities that are by-products of some of the other foods we eat. The insoluble fibers act more like a gentle scouring agent, loosening the waste materials that might tend to cling to the cell walls in your system.

The best fiber for your body is whole grain food, like bran. That's right, the lowly bran muffin or bran breakfast cereal is great for you. Whole wheat bran is excellent for your system. Among the best cereals on the market are plain Cream of Wheat, Grapenuts, Nutri-grain, Quaker Oats (Quick or Old-Fashioned, or even plain instant), Ralston, shredded wheat, Total, and the "Breakfast of Champions," Wheaties.

Although you will be getting healthful fiber from rice and whole wheat bread, the milling methods used on these foods removes some of the helpful qualities of the fiber. Don't rely on them alone.

Other foods with fiber include kidney beans, blackberries, parsnips, peas, apples, pears, plums, broccoli, white potatoes, squash, green beans, strawberries, tomatoes, and zucchini.

In addition to helping prevent cancer, fiber foods (the soluble forms such as fruits and vegetables) help control your cholesterol and blood-sugar levels.

Beef

There is a connection between fats and cancer, and beef is high in fat. Beyond that, however, there is some suspicion that beef consumption contributes to bowel cancer. For example, the people of Scotland consume more beef than the people of England. About 20 percent more, in fact. The incidence of bowel cancer among the Scots is almost exactly 20 percent higher than among the English. Other statistical evidence follows this pattern.

Whether or not it is the fatty nature of beef that is responsible, or something in the way beef is treated or cooked, is not yet known.

Hamburger

When chopped meat is grilled on metal over 300 degrees Fahrenheit, mutagens are produced. These substances can cause genetic change. Most mutagens tend to promote cancer, which makes hamburgers a suspected cancer-causing food, depending on the method of preparation (broiling usually does not produce mutagens, and meat that is lightly cooked and eaten rare is also usually free of mutagens). The meat itself isn't the question (although the fat content is still a problem), but avoid grilling or frying meat to the point of charring.

Nitrites

When the makers of baby food voluntarily removed nitrites from their products in the 1970s, that should have been the signal to us all to avoid these food additives. Both potassium nitrite and sodium nitrite can combine with the natural chemicals in your stomach to form a cancer-causing agent called nitrosamine.

Nitrites are still used as an additive (to make products look more like raw meat) in the manufacture of such things as bologna, bacon, cured meats, smoke-cured products, hot dogs, meat spread, sausages, spiced ham, and so forth.

Unfortunately, nitrites are the best known means of preventing the growth of botulism in certain products, which is at least a more valid reason for using them than simple cosmetic concerns. Still, it might be best to avoid the problem as much as possible by avoiding these types of foods as much as possible.

To give you an idea of how I act in this area, I used to enjoy a meal of hot dogs about three times a month. Now, I eat one at the ball park about once every two months or so. Once in a while my wife and I will eat one apiece at home. And that's it. The point is to cut down on your consumption until more is known.

Bacon

The meat from the back and sides of hogs isn't called bacon until it has been salted, smoked, and colored with nitrites. The nitrites combine with naturally occurring amines to form nitrosamines, which are known to cause cancer.

Meat processors are currently required to keep formations of nitrosamines to less than 10 parts per billion, but they are allowed to do it by adding chemical derivatives of vitamin C, which block nitrosamine formations.

It's no wonder there are so many new bacon substitutes on the market.

Sunlight

The phrase "thick skinned" usually means insensitive to other's hints or insults but in this case it means the literal measurement of your skin layer. Some people can withstand more ultraviolet light from the sun than others.

Your skin pigmentation is also a factor. Usually, the fairer the skin color, the more sensitive to the ultraviolet light.

In any case, prolonged and repeated tanning produces more than dry, wrinkled skin. It also contributes to skin cancer.

It is odd that we have done a flip-flop as regards a tanned skin. In the early part of this century, the only people with tanned skin were laborers whose menial work kept them exposed to the sun's rays. The well-to-do were able to keep themselves protected from the sun. Nowadays, when the majority of workers are in offices, only those with excess time on their hands can "work on their tans." Thus it has become some sort of badge of the wealthy leisure class to be suntanned. We know that anyone can lie out on his or her driveway during the weekend and soak up some rays, but somehow our culture still equates a tan with a healthy and wealthy person.

Just keep in mind that a little sun goes a long way. Besides, what's wrong with being fair skinned? What woman would not enjoy hearing Christopher Marlowe's "Oh, thou art fairer than the evening air/Clad in the beauty of a thousand stars"?

Water

In addition to what you learned in the chapter on water, you should be aware that there are some concerns that unpurified water may contain suspected carcinogens. A National Academy of Sciences investigation into the drinking water of American cities discovered twenty-two compounds present in our water that are either known or suspected carcinogens. The amounts were very small—perhaps too small to be cancer-causing in humans. But the decision to rely on city-supplied water for oral use must be weighed against the possible risks. If the possibility of cancer isn't meaningful enough, go back to Chapter 10 for both the good and bad news about water.

17

A Few Words About Alcohol

EVERYTHING you need to know about drinking can be summed up in one word. Don't.

Now let's be realistic

Okay, I admit it: I drink. Beer, mostly, but I have been known to have wine and the occasional gin and tonic (except when in England, when I happily switch to gin and lime).

My wife bought me Michael Jackson's wonderful book *The Pocket Guide to Beer* and we've been seeking out the various highly rated beers of the world whenever circumstances (read: personal financial conditions) allow. Yet our most intense drinking bout consisted of one wild night in which we had three beers. (With the low-alcohol beers, we might get up to four beers.)

Why this moderation? It's certainly not for lack of opportunity, as we both work in the advertising business.

Well, for one thing, we both experienced what it's like to have too much to drink. I never want to repeat the hell of that next morning. The high caloric content of drinks is another reason.

The primary reason, however, has to do with breaking the concentration needed for The Ego Diet. Alcohol makes you do, say, and eat things you probably wouldn't otherwise. Because of this, alcohol is dangerous quite apart from the risk of getting too inebriated to drive safely.

What happens when you drink?

Different things happen to different people. Some get sad. Some get happy. Some get much too happy. There are boring, maudlin, hostile, and hysterical drunks. A few people kill themselves. A few others kill others.

All this happens because of changes in the brain. In general, you can say that the refinements of civilization are stripped away by alcohol.

Here's how:

The booze you swallow gets into your bloodstream and the alcohol eventually enters your brain. It seeps through the small blood vessels called capillaries and into the nerve cells of your brain.

Now, there's a chemical reaction inside your head. First, it affects your alertness control, called the reticular formation. This, in turn, deadens the cerebral cortex, the most important brain center in humans. By deadens, I don't mean to suggest it is blocked off or blacked out. Your organizational ability is impaired. And while ideas may speed through your brain faster and faster, they will not come out making much sense.

As the alcohol infects your brain, you lose control of your motor-speech functions, your muscle coordination, your motor activity, and your vision. Obviously, one drink will not bring the normal human body to the state of collapse, yet all the areas I've mentioned are affected, and the degree depends on the amount of alcohol consumed, the amount of food in the stomach, the tolerance of the body, and the size of the body in question.

Okay, but what's the "bottom line"?

Some people don't want to know what alcohol does to their body, much less to their brain. They just want to skip to the bottom line: what's so bad about the things alcohol does?

Basically, alcohol is a depressant.

"But wait a minute," a young man said to me at a meeting. "It may depress you, but it makes me feel happy."

Wrong. You may think you feel happy, but what is really happening is you're becoming uninhibited. The alcohol simply removes some barriers that you've put up against your more antisocial instincts.

Remember how the id keeps whispering in your ear that you should "go for it" and heed your baser feelings? But your superego (which is basically like your conscience) keeps telling you to behave yourself, conform, go easy, and don't rock the boat. It's your ego that judges the correct balance between the two, based on what's happening in your own mind and body and what appears to be happening with your relationships with others around you. Alcohol tends to remove the edge from all three, leaving you rudderless and without bearings.

If you're feeling sad but have been trying to hide it, alcohol may bring on the morose, feeling-sorry-for-yourself blahs. Or it may lead you to tears.

If you've been under pressure at home or office, alcohol may make you "forget" the problems you're having so you can relax. Unfortunately, people like to go farther than this (or cannot judge when or where to stop) and the result is overcompensation—you begin whooping it up. And, depending on the circumstances, you will make a large or small fool of yourself. Because you may well be in the company of other fools, who've been drinking and who can't tell that you're acting like an idiot, they might applaud your stupid behavior. At best, you might safely let off a little steam this way. Often, however, you read about barroom brawls that began when two people disagreed on how the other should be whooping or hollering.

Either way—if you get sad or glad, or even just somewhere in between—the alcohol is bringing you down, depressing your brainpower, and hurting your system.

"I'm drinking to, uh . . ."

The fact that the alcoholic depression tends to make them "forget" their troubles is an attraction to some people. The old joke about the man in the bar saying he's "only drinking to forget," but not being able to remember what he's trying to forget or even how long he's been trying, does have some basis in reality.

Still, whatever it is that the alcohol has pushed to the background areas of your mind will probably be around the next morning. This will make you either face up to them or go out and "forget" again. But you'll find that you need a little more alcohol to get the fog to enshroud your brain this time. And, lo and behold, the problems will still be there the following day.

Assuming you don't mind the horrible feelings of queasiness in the stomach and the throbbing in the head, you then might try to forget again that evening, after work. Or, as some people in advertising do, at lunch.

Eventually, you get into a terrible pattern of drinking, sobering up, drinking, sobering up, and so forth. Meanwhile, you end up barely coping with your job. You limp around work trying to function on one or two cylinders instead of with full power.

A confession

One evening I got drunk. Good and drunk. And I "forgot about all my troubles." In fact, I forgot about almost everything.

I was invited to see an advance screening of a new film about teenagers and their favorite hang-out, a drive-in restaurant. As part of the promotional activities for the film, everyone at the screening was also invited to a private party to be held at Tiny Naylor's, a popular drive-in nearby (and scene of many sequences in the film).

It was great. Tables with cloth covers and padded chairs were set up all around the drive-in, while various classic cars and custom hot rods were on display all over the parking lot in between the tables. Adding to the decadently exclusive nature of the affair was the crowd of fans straining against the iron barricades surrounding the restaurant and parking lot. These antiriot structures had been towed into place by the police to keep our private party private—although the people crushed onto the sidewalk could see us clearly, they could not get in.

Free food and drink were in plentiful supply, so I began enjoying myself. A lot. I chatted with my friends, and had a drink. I chatted with some of the film's actors, and had a drink. I went over to the barricades and chatted with some of the public, and had a drink. For no reason at all I had a drink. I had become stoned. Blotto. Soused. Pie-eyed. I may or may not have been happy, but I suspect not. It's a moot point, because I couldn't really feel much of anything. I am extremely fortunate I have friends who care about me or I might have been involved in an automobile accident while trying to get home. The rest of the evening was a blur.

Getting up the next morning was an exercise in, well, exercise. I could have used a crowbar to help pry my head off the pillow. Standing up was a dizzying feat. Walking was a major advancement in latent motor skills. Any sound louder than two pillows brushing together sent ice-cold shivers skipping up and down my spine. I took two antiseasickness tablets just to back the car out of the driveway. The journey to the business district was a heart-stopping session of "Dodge 'em Cars"—with real cars.

At work, a vile cacophony of putrid phony-music noises filled the elevator. Of course, it did that every day, but never before at the volume level of a jetliner in an echo chamber.

The building's air conditioning system created an intense rushing sound that entered my ears at different times and at different pitches no matter which way I turned my head. The only comfortable way to move was with both hands clamped over my ears—not easy when you're carrying a briefcase, rumpled sportcoat, and morning newspaper. As I slumped slowly down the hallway, I was reminded of the sequences in the film *2001: A Space Odyssey* in which the astronauts put on their space suits and heavy breathing filled the sound track.

After trudging ten or fifteen miles I finally reached my office. I swung my arms forward, letting go of briefcase, coat, and paper at the uppermost point on the arc, then quickly put my hands back over my ears so I wouldn't hear them hit the floor. I went on another trek, in search of coffee.

Office coffee is pretty poor even under the best of circumstances. That day, it tasted like watered-down mud mixed with vinegar. I poured it down my gullet.

Yet another pilgrimage through the tortuous hallways to my cubicle. Perhaps it was the light shooting through the open curtains that blinded me. Perhaps I had a synapse lapse somewhere in the cranium. I'll never know what caused it, but I scored a billiard off the filing cabinet and the edge of the desk before careening into my chair: bump-clunk-plop.

It was a singularly unproductive day for me. The business may have hummed along, generating another ten million dollars or so, but I was a closed file through all of it. I sat and stared and contemplated the vast number of quicker, easier, and more attractive ways to die I could have chosen.

Never again

I said it that day. Often. And I've lived up to that promise. I will not allow myself to drink past the point of losing appreciable control over what I'm saying or doing.

It may not be chic, but I've done something that helps me prove to myself whether or not I had enough to drink. I simply recite some schoolyard phrase that requires a bit of speech dexterity. The old standby is "Peter Piper picked a peck of pickled peppers." But you can also use "How much wood would a woodchuck chuck if a woodchuck would chuck wood?" You can also perform the classic police test in which you close your eyes, hold your arms straight out from your shoulders and, bending them at the elbows, attempt to gently touch the tip of your nose alternately with each hand. I find that trying to pat yourself on the belly while simultaneously moving your other hand in a circular motion above your head works wonders for getting you to put down your next drink in favor of coffee, soft drinks, juice, or water.

In case you missed it

On the off chance you didn't get the reinforcement of the public service message subtly woven into the preceding story, let me spell it out for you: If you drink, don't drive.

Alcohol is involved with about 50 percent of all traffic deaths.

Alcohol misuse accounts for about 200,000 deaths a year in the United States alone. Don't get behind the wheel of a car when your brain is befuddled by booze.

"But I need a drink"

Nonsense. Only someone addicted to alcohol "needs" a drink, and then only to avoid getting an attack of delirium tremens (the D.T.'s).

You may feel as if you need to be dulled out by alcohol, but this is just a state of mind. More than likely you're just being lazy—too lazy to simply take the time necessary to calm down and deal with your problems in a rational manner. You're looking to alcohol for an escape from reality. You want alcohol to smash down your fears and frustrations. This is probably true in 90 percent of the times that you have a minor craving for a drink. I believe this because I go through many of the same problems you do, and I get the same cravings.

People have told me very earnestly that they "can't make it through the day without having a drink" at lunch or at some other point during their workday. Hogwash. They are lying to themselves because they enjoy getting a shot of booze during working hours.

"If I can't calm my nerves," one man told me, "I'll lose my job." He claimed he takes a drink before going in to see his boss. Naturally, he uses some sort of spray or mint to cover those alcoholic fumes that engulfed his tongue, teeth, and mouth after drinking.

Having had a very obtuse boss at one point, I can sympathize with the desire for dulling your wits before visiting the great man. Many times I've had to bite my lip in order to keep from saying something that would show I was aware of the load of horse manure being shoveled around the executive suite. All that means, however, is exercising a little self-control. (Oh all right, maybe a lot of self-control.)

If you're working for people who aren't brighter than you are, go out and find some smarter people. Make them prove their smarts by hiring you. In the meantime, keep your mouth shut and your mind open. Perhaps you can find a way to suggest an idea in just the right way so that the person in charge will pick it up and make it his or her own idea. That will make working at your present place a bit better in the short run, and perhaps you won't need to look for excuses to drink.

I don't know of too many people who enjoy being around others who drink too much. You probably don't like it, so you shouldn't put other people through it on your account. That guy who drank before seeing his boss wasn't a fun fellow to be around. He said he wished he could get a different job. I asked him how his search for one was going. He said he wasn't looking! "Why in heaven's name not?" I asked. Why would he put up with the terrors of the current job and not even try finding another one?

Then it hit me. He was the kind of a person who would rather take a drink than face up to a problem. To some people, that makes him a regular guy, a guy whose problems justify his being a two-fisted drinker. To me, it makes him a wimp.

"How can I drink more now than I could before?"

You probably realize that larger people have a greater capacity for alcohol than smaller people. With more blood to carry the alcohol, more cells to be affected, and a larger stomach—all else being equal—the person with the higher body weight will fall down drunk after everyone else has passed out. If this is of some importance or gains you stature among your particular social set, then by all means close this book and go out and get as fat as Jabba the Hutt.

Still, the question about the amount of alcohol consumed is important. You may have noticed that you're drinking more in order to get the same effect. Or you've seen that two people of similar size may drink widely differing amounts of liquor with the big drinker getting no more and no less tipsy than the little sipper. The difference is in the tolerance each has built up within his or her body.

The first time you have a drink, your body is totally unprepared for the alcohol. Thus, you don't need much of the stuff to feel a real buzz in your brain. As you get accustomed to having a bit of wine at lunch or dinner, your body is adjusting to the impurities now coursing through your system on a daily basis. With moderation, this is no big deal. Carried to excess, you can actually train your digestive system to assimilate more and more alcohol and do it better and better (in the sense of being efficient at cleaning out your innards). Then, you need more and more alcohol to get the same feeling of tipsiness (or whatever state you're aiming for).

Your liver, the largest organ in your body, acts as a sort of filtering agent for the alcohol you pour into your stomach. Although not by any means the only vital organ affected by your use of liquor, it will serve as an illustration of the importance of not overdoing it when dealing with alcohol. When you drink, you are forcing your liver to work overtime. The more you ask it to work for you on these "recreational" activities, the less it can work for you in warding off disease. The more you tax it with liquor, the less it has to help keep you strong and healthy. Sure, your liver gets used to having to flush out your body more than before, but why wear it out in the process. For that matter, your whole body gets used to alcohol. So does your brain—do you intend to wear it out, too?

Look at it this way: if you experience a greater effect from less alcohol when your system is not used to drink, just think how much fun you'll have when you do decide to have that occasional cocktail.

Your introduction to alcohol

Chances are, you first encountered alcohol under less than ideal circumstances. Most people do.

It happens at parties. Or out behind the supermarket. Or in someone's car. Almost always in a situation where you don't have any control and are subject to peer pressure.

If you're lucky to have had parents who cared very much about you, they introduced you to alcohol in such a way as to avoid your having a rough experience. If you care about your children, you'll do the same for them. Do it in your home, away from any social pressure. Make certain no one else is around to apply peer pressure. Don't ask anything of your children except an open mind. You'll help them a lot by revealing that it is possible to use a small amount of alcohol in a quiet, contemplative setting that doesn't require them to entertain anyone or drive anywhere.

By making it a pleasurable, low-key occasion—just what alcohol itself should represent—you'll be greatly increasing the odds of your children treating alcohol with respect later in life.

Let's look at calories

Alcohol is fattening. Not for nothing has the term "beer belly" been bandied about by observers of middle-aged men. While it is assumed that beer is less likely to cause drunkenness, because it contains less alcohol than mixed drinks or cocktails, the problem is that people feel free to have lots of it. Just because you keep going to the rest room doesn't mean the alcohol isn't staying in your body . . . along with the calories.

A mixed drink or several beers, when added to your normal day's intake of food, might account for as much as a 10 percent increase in your caloric total for that day. Here are some average calorie counts for several popular drinks:

Southern Comfort—240 (2 ounces)
80 proof whiskey—130 (2 ounces)
90 proof whiskey—150 (2 ounces)
Beer—150 (12 ounces)
Gin and tonic—190 (8 ounces)
Irish coffee—270 (8 ounces)
Margarita—200 (4 ounces)
Martini—200 (4 ounces)
Screwdriver—175 (6 ounces)

Of course, these can be higher depending on the way you or your bartender fixes the drinks. When in doubt, I took the low average. That's a hell of a shove down the road that leads to obesity . . . especially when you consider that all those calories come in what amounts to a few ounces of water, juice, mixer, and booze.

Alcohol and cancer

As you've already seen, they are related. If you drink a lot, you are statistically more likely to contract cancer than people who refrain from drinking. Misuse of alcohol will lead to a traffic accident sooner than it will lead to cancer, true enough, but that's only because cancer often takes thirty years to develop, leaving you plenty of time to get into several auto collisions. The fact remains that the use of alcohol is associated with cancer of the liver, esophagus, and mouth. Primary liver cancer is attributed to alcohol consumption almost exclusively.

Alcohol and other ailments

One of the ten leading causes of death in the United States is cirrhosis, or fibrosis of the liver, in which the fibers inside the liver grow to the point of cutting off the functioning of the liver. There is no cure. One of the primary causes of cirrhosis is the consumption of alcohol.

Some neurological disorders—malfunctions within the human nervous system—are directly attributable to alcohol use and misuse. And remember, since the U.S. Surgeon General defines a problem drinker as anyone who drinks to intoxication at least once a month, misuse of alcohol may not involve as much drinking as you think.

Alcohol versus nutrition

If you drink heavily, you may lose your appetite for the very foods you need most: those containing essential vitamins and minerals.

Deficiencies occur not only because of the drinker's tendency to bypass many good foods, but because alcohol alters how your body absorbs and uses some nutrients. Even moderate use of alcohol can affect the amount of niacin and thiamine your body receives. Both of these vitamins are essential in metabolism.

No answer

There are two questions that are frequently asked about alcohol that have their genesis in American folklore. That's the charitable way of saying old wive's tales.

The first question concerns the use of alcohol by women who are pregnant. Whenever I have been asked if some alcohol consumption is good for pregnant women, invariably the questioner lets it be known that he or she feels the answer is "yes." Unfortunately, this answer is partially correct, which can lead to problems. Some pregnancies, under some circumstances, may be helped by a regulated use of alcohol. This does not mean you should run out and begin lapping up the stuff to try discovering if you're one of these special cases. Ask your doctor. The old wive's tale has it that *every* pregnancy is helped by alcohol, and this is simply not true.

The second question concerns alcohol use in general. Because the 1979 U.S. Surgeon General's Report stated that "One or two drinks daily appear to cause no harm in adults," many people wonder if having a couple of cocktails each day is really so bad. Well, judge for yourself. Do you need the calories? Can you afford to handle the tipsiness? Do you intend to drive immediately afterward? Do you mind the cost? Can you still remain on your healthy diet? Is your liver strong?

Consider, too, that there are great differences in body types, personality types, body weights and sizes, physical tolerance levels, and so forth. You might be fine having two drinks a day for the rest of your very long, very healthy life. Or, you might be pushing your luck when you have one single drink—if you have that drink at the wrong time.

The choice is completely yours, but nowhere in the Surgeon General's Report is anything other than moderation with alcohol recommended.

If you do drink . . .

In *Mark Twain Tonight*, Hal Holbrook's celebrated stage portrayal of the humorist and author, there is a lovely adaptation of something Twain wrote about alcohol in "Letters to Satan" from *Europe and Else-*

where. Twain is being admonished by his doctor because of excessive drinking, and Twain replies that he only drinks "as a preventative of toothache. (Pause) I've never had the toothache. (Pause) And I don't ever intend to have it."

Well, for those of us who also plan never to have the toothache, there are some practical suggestions to compensate for the intake of alcohol:

 ► Eat nutritious foods that are low in calories (lean meat, fish, poultry, fruits, vegetables, and grains).
 ► Make sure you have a variety of foods in your diet (to avoid having your body miss out on any essential nutrients).
 ► Avoid an excess of cholesterol, fat, or saturated fat.
 ► Choose foods with fiber (see Chapter 16).
 ► Avoid sugar.
 ► Avoid too much sodium.

Flush your system

By drinking water after drinking alcohol, you'll help your body cleanse your digestive system and accomplish two additional things. First, you'll delay your having a second drink. And second, you'll be filling up on something other than alcohol at precisely the point at which the alcohol is having its greatest effect—thereby prolonging the sensation of having a drink without actually having any additional alcohol.

Overindulging

The standard, cliché remedy for drinking too much is to pour coffee, hot and black, down your throat. While I cannot dispute the fact that the caffeine in the coffee does seem to help some people in dire straits, in most other instances the action of coffee is largely myth. We believe coffee will help us sober up and so it does help. In reality, water or fruit juice may be better for you.

What about the "hair of the dog" treatment? This quaint saying, which comes from John Heywood's *Proverbs* (first printed in 1546), means that a small amount of the same drink that caused so much trouble the night before should be sipped during the morning after. The theory is that if we have "a hair of the dog that bit us," as the saying goes, we'll be cured. Like the idea of catching birds simply by sprinkling salt on their tails, it has no basis in fact.

Maintain your high self-image

If you control alcohol instead of the other way around, common sense will see you through most situations. With what you now know about alcohol, you can easily choose the best course of action for you, based on your current diet and your eating plans for the day.

If you take a drink, keep a mental picture of your ideal self in front of you. Or, you may find it more helpful to keep a mental picture of your role model in your head. Either way, use the very act of sipping your drink as a "trigger" to recall the image.

With the right picture in your mind's eye, you can use alcohol wisely and safely—and maintain your healthy diet.

18

A Few Words About Vitamins

THE television set is on one Saturday morning. In between the old Tom & Jerry cartoons and the Adventures of Space Cowboy & His Intergalactic Star Fighters comes an animated commercial for chewable children's vitamins.

The pace of the commercial is even faster than the zowie-powie-blam-boom effects during the shows. Like the programming, the commercial is brightly colored and loudly orchestrated with sophisticated mixtures of traditional instruments and special sound effects.

In the spot, which lasts only thirty seconds, a talking bottle of vitamins flies through outer space, zooms across a city, comes in the window of a child's home, ejects a glowing chewy vitamin into Mom's hands, pats both Mom and the child on the back after the child has chomped the tablet, and metamorphoses into its real self as it appears affixed to a piece of cardboard in the supermarket. All of which is quite entertaining, of course, and certainly free of misrepresentation as far as I'm concerned. What is a bit disturbing is the effect the vitamin tablet appears to have on the child. He smiles, glows, and grows bigger. He also picks himself up off his chair and scoots rapidly out of the house and back in again in an instant.

Contrary to belief, vitamins do not produce any energy in your body.

They do have a crucial function, just the same, for without vitamins, your metabolism—the converting of food into energy—could not take place.

What do vitamins do?

Most vitamins help the enzymes in your body as they react with food to extract the fuel and nutrients and discard the waste materials. Some vitamins are catalysts, meaning they speed up some enzymatic or oxidative reactions. Without this effect, the chemical reactions inside your body would take too long to do any good, or they would require a much higher temperature than your body can provide. Other vitamins act as forerunners of enzymes, preparing the way for the reactions that are to come.

Certain vitamins have specific targets in your body: some will help strengthen your bones; some will help your tissues; and some help your body absorb food in the intestine.

Where do we get vitamins?

Almost every vitamin needed by your body comes inside the food in the basic food groups: meat, dairy products, fruits and vegetables, and grains. Some vitamins are created inside your body: they are synthesized (created through the reaction of two or more compounds) by bacterial action inside your large intestine. From there, these vitamins are absorbed into the bloodstream.

Is it wrong to take vitamin tablets?

It isn't wrong to take them as long as you don't rely on the tablets to supply the majority of vitamins to your body. Vitamin tablets are actually *vitamin supplements*—to be taken, as the name implies, only to supplement your normal intake of vitamins in the food you eat.

It is a mistake to assume, as some people do, that taking vitamin tablets replaces the need to eat vegetables or some other food every day.

Vitamin deficiencies

Ever since sailors first went on long voyages, it has been known that some diseases are associated with the lack of fresh foods. Various methods have been used to compensate for this lack. English sailors were required to drink lime juice during long voyages, which is why they became known as limeys.

There are six primary reasons for vitamin deficiency:

► Low intake of foods with vitamins
► Failure of the body to absorb vitamins
► Liver disease
► The body's increased demand for vitamins, so the normal amount isn't enough
► Deterioration of the gastrointestinal tract
► A lack of the proper reactive substance in the body

Some of these are rare, and none of them are associated with healthy individuals, but others are easy to fall into without some care in your planning of your diet.

Obviously, if you don't eat foods from the primary food groups you'll be making yourself a prime candidate for vitamin deficiency and the many diseases that follow from it. By eating at least one food item from each food group each day, you'll be helping your body get its natural vitamins.

A low intake of the proper foods often results from a special diet being used to treat an allergy, hypertension, or a peptic ulcer, or from a restricted diet during the recuperation period following an illness or operation. In all these cases, a physician is usually carefully monitoring the patient's progress so that adequate steps can be taken to compensate for the body's lack of vitamins.

When there is a low intake of proper foods due to a crash diet or fad diet, often no doctor is available. This is because the people who are likely to put themselves on a foolish fad or crash diet are the type of people who will not heed a physician's advice about weight loss. People using the slow, measured, and sensible weight-loss methods of The Ego Diet are more willing to seek medical advice, and physicians are much more receptive to this plan.

When an individual has difficulty absorbing vitamins, most likely it is due to one of three things. First, the person may be vomiting or suffering from prolonged diarrhea so that the body doesn't have sufficient time to grab onto the vitamins in the food. Second, there may be an absence of bile salts in the intestine (they must be present for the absorption of fat-soluble vitamins). Or, third, the person may be using mineral oil as a laxative. (Excessive use of low-calorie salad dressings may have this same effect—the mineral oil in these types of dressings carry off the needed fat-soluble vitamins during elimination.) In all these cases, see your doctor; and avoid the dangerous crash-diet practices that cause trouble.

In liver disease, your body fails to create forerunners to vitamins or fails to store vitamins. See your doctor if you are not already under a physician's care.

There are times when your body needs more vitamins than usual—if you are suffering from some fevers, for example. Other examples include pregnancy and lactation (the formation of milk in the breast for the feeding of the newborn).

If you suffer from the breakdown of the gastrointestinal tract, you should be under a doctor's care. It is possible that this may be a side effect of a cure for some other ailment, because there are some antibiotics that prevent bacterial action in the gut, which can lead to the intestinal breakdown.

There are certain amino acids that must be present in your body if the proper chemical reactions are to take place and vitamins are to be delivered to the ideal spots. Without this, vitamin deficiency will certainly follow. Again, expert advice is required.

Fat-soluble vitamins

Vitamin A: it helps in growth and in the maintenance of your mucous membranes. Without it, bones will not grow, vision is impaired, the skin becomes rough and dry, and night blindness affects you. *Vitamin A is found in yellow fruits, yellow vegetables, and dark green leafy vegetables.*

Vitamin D: helps in the calcification of bones and in the absorption of such minerals as calcium in the intestine. Without it, the young suffer rickets—bones get soft and fragile, joints become enlarged, teeth do not form properly, and the legs may become bowed. In adults, a lack of D leads to a softening of bones, which in turn may lead to deformities of the spine, pelvis, or legs. In addition, fractures are quite frequent. *Plant vitamin D and animal vitamin D are produced in the body when plant and animal sterols are acted on by ultraviolet light (as in sunshine). Getting outdoors for a few moments each day is a good idea (as is eating properly).*

Vitamin K: helps in the coagulation of the blood. Without it, hemorrhaging may result. *Vitamin K is present in fish meal, pork liver, spinach, and cabbage.*

Vitamin E: protects vitamins A and D and helps prevent the breakdown of red blood cells. Without it, children may suffer from cystic fibrosis. Little is known about effects in adults except that vitamins A and D may not always remain in your system without vitamin E being present. *Vitamin E is in wheat germ oil, lettuce, and green leafy vegetables.*

Water-soluble vitamins

Thiamine: helps in metabolism, and contributes to your mental health and well-being. Without it, you can suffer from anorexia, vomiting, weakness, impaired coordination, and even beriberi, a disease that affects the nerves, heart, and digestion. *You find thiamine in dry peas, beans, soybeans, yeast, whole wheat bread, avocados, dried prunes, figs, pork, milk, cheese, pecans, and Brazil nuts.*

Riboflavin: helps in metabolism, in obtaining energy from food. Without it, you could suffer inflammation of the tongue, mouth, and skin. *Riboflavin is synthesized by all green plants and is also found in yeast, kidney, liver, and wheat germ.*

Niacin: helps enzymes, aids in the synthesis of fats and the utilization of glucose for energy. Without it, a number of different kinds of lesions (harmful change in the structure of an organ) may result. Even worse, pellagra may result—pellagra is known as the disease of the four D's: dementia, dermatitis, diarrhea, and death. *Good sources of niacin include lean meat, fish, kidney, liver, heart, yeast, peanuts, peas, beans, and wheat germ.*

Pantothenic acid: helps in metabolism. Without it, people experience personality changes, fatigue, somnolence, insomnia, a staggering walk, and some gastrointestinal problems. *It is found in liver, eggs, yeast, and is formed by bacteria in the intestine (provided the right foods are present).*

B_6: needed for chemical actions involving amino acids. Without it, excessive dryness sets in around the eyes, eyebrows, and mouth. Also, your ability to form antibodies is impaired. *You get it in foods containing other B-complex vitamins, like rice, wheat germ, yeast, egg yolk, and seeds.*

Biotin: needed for reactions involving enzymes. There is some doubt about the effects of biotin shortage, because it rarely occurs on its own. Suffice it to say that it contributes to the good of other vitamins and a lack of it leads to other vitamin deficiencies. *It is found in kidney, liver, yeast, molasses, milk, egg yolk, nuts, vegetables, and grains.*

Folic acid: helps in metabolism. Without it, diarrhea, anemia, lesions, and inflammation of the tongue may result. *Sources include leafy green vegetables and yeast.*

B_{12}: helps in metabolism. Without it, you could suffer from anemia. B_{12} *is found in kidney, liver, animal muscle, and fish muscle.*

Inositol: it prevents the buildup of fat and cholesterol in the liver. *You get it in seeds, roots, and tubers like the potato.*

Ascorbic acid (vitamin C): it helps in the production of supporting tissues, bones, teeth, and connective tissues. Without it, scurvy may result. This produces a loosening of teeth, soreness of gums, bleeding, painful joints, and anemia. *You get vitamin C in citric fruits and fresh vegetables like turnip greens and broccoli.*

Are vitamins stored in the body?

Some are, some aren't. Vitamins A, D, E, and K are retained in your body for some period of time, but others must be replenished every day if you are to remain healthy.

It was once believed that water-soluble vitamins would be stored in the body up to the proper amount needed, but that an "overdose" of water-soluble vitamins would be "washed away" by elimination of water by the body. Now, it appears this is not so. Beware of diets or cures that suggest massive ingestion of any vitamin. This can lead to a toxic effect not unlike poisoning.

Vitamins and sex

There is a "lover's diet" on the market that, despite its nomenclature, is actually quite healthy. The diet for a healthy sex life is quite close to the diet for a healthy life, period. As such, it fits in perfectly with The Ego Diet.

This "sexy diet" is, like The Ego Diet, low in fats, salt, sugar, white flour, and traditional "bad foods" such as coffee, doughnuts, cake, chocolate, and so on. It is high in grain, vegetables, lean meats, fruit, nuts, seeds, and fish.

As you can see from that list, most of the necessary vitamins would be ingested with the good food. Still, the lover's diet claims that a vitamin supplement is necessary. The advocates of this sexy diet recommend taking vitamin E and vitamin C in tablet or capsule form, although even they recognize the value of simply increasing your intake of foods high in these vitamins.

They call vitamin E "the sex vitamin." Of the benefits listed by these happy folk, the main ones are prevention of inflammation of the prostate (the muscular gland at the base of the bladder in males) and inflammation of the vagina in women.

The benefits of eating the right foods are so good in and of themselves, you'll probably feel so much more full of life that your sexual activities will just naturally increase and improve. Is this due to the vitamins? Perhaps. If this is what makes you want to eat the healthy foods, then think of sexual escapades when confronted by chocolate cake, and eat a carrot instead (rabbit food, you know).

Natural food tranquilizers

Some foods seem to have a calming effect on many people. You might want to try some of the foods mentioned in this section and see if you don't feel that your nerves are less jangled and your blood is less likely to boil at the vagaries of life.

Lecithin, pronounced "less-uh-thin," is a nutrient that is extracted from soybeans. You can purchase it in powdered form or in tablets or capsules. While it has not had an effect on me, I have spoken to many people who swear by it, so it may have something to do with your natural metabolism rate or other factors involving your diet. Some people find that lecithin not only soothes their nerves. but also combats sexual dysfunction and debilitating fatigue. Since it is not a chemical additive but a natural food product, it cannot hurt you when taken in the recommended doses listed on the bottle.

Dolomite is the name given to the combination of the minerals calcium and magnesium. It, too, is supposed to calm your nerves. There may be some basis in fact for this claim, as a low calcium blood count has been often associated with irritability. And magnesium does help control blood cholesterol, so perhaps dolomite pills will help control nervousness.

Almost all of the calcium in your body—about 99 percent—is in your teeth and bones, but that other 1 percent must come from the food you eat. It's better if it comes from milk, but if you cannot have milk, dolomite might be a good substitute. Ask your doctor.

Powdered brewer's yeast (which is not the same as uncooked baker's yeast) is almost all protein, with no sugar, fat, or starch to speak of. It is a good source of B vitamins, and does seem to exert a soothing influence on some people.

Yogurt is another tranquil food, and it is very good for you. Even the frozen yogurt (which contains sugar) is not bad for you. It helps digestion, provides protein, helps cleanse your breath, and it can help you calm down. It works for me, so I have no problem claiming it as a natural food tranquilizer.

The urge to snack can be overpowering, but putting some nuts and carob-covered raisins into a cup of fruit-at-the-bottom yogurt will help you both at the snack time and when you sit down for a meal. It you eat a cup of yogurt a half hour prior to your meal, you'll eat much less than you'd planned . . . and you'll have added something very healthy to your diet.

Some people also claim fructose is a natural tranquilizer that helps you get through snack times. It is fruit sugar, as opposed to refined (white) sugar. It is more natural, and also seems to calm you down, even if you put it in coffee. The only problem I have with fructose is that its sweet taste sometimes makes me crave the sweet taste of foods with refined sugar, and that is very dangerous. You'll have to try it and see if it replaces your craving for other sugary substances, or if it merely adds to it.

Space-age vitamins

Many books and films have shown astronauts taking their meals in tablet form or from tubes. Much is made of the tablets having "the same number of vitamins and minerals" as other meals.

Well, this may be true someday. But for right now, don't think you can get your vitamins from a tube or a tablet. They are found in foods —good, healthy foods.

VITAMIN AND NUTRIENT GUIDE

Fresh Vegetables	Vitamins A	B	C	Fiber	Iron	Magnesium	Calcium
Asparagus	X		X		X		
Lima beans		X		X	X		
Beets				X			
Broccoli	X	X	X	X	X	X	
Cabbage			X	X			
Carrots	X			X			
Cauliflower			X	X			
Celery				X			
Corn				X			
Mushrooms				X			
Peas		X		X	X		
Potatoes		X	X	X			
Spinach	X	X	X	X	X	X	X
Summer squash	X			X			

VITAMIN AND NUTRIENT GUIDE

Fresh Fruit	Vitamins A	B	C	Fiber	Iron	Magnesium	Calcium
Apples				X			
Apricots	X			X			
Bananas		X		X		X	
Blueberries				X	X		
Cherries			X				
Grapefruit			X				
Grapes			X				
Nectarines	X			X			
Oranges			X	X			
Peaches	X			X			
Pears				X			
Plums			X	X			
Raspberries			X	X	X		
Strawberries			X	X	X		
Watermelon			X				

19

Foods That Fool You

SO you think you know your food. Well, you know enough of the basics to agree with every one of the following general statements:

> Salads are good.
> Desserts are bad.
> Lean meats (like veal) are good.
> Fatty meats (like steak and hamburger) are bad.
> Baked or broiled foods are better than pan-fried or deep-fried.
> Fresh foods are better than canned.

You probably knew most of that before you even picked up this book, but these facts should certainly have been solidly reinforced by now. After the first eighteen chapters, you probably know a lot more about your approach to food in general and your reaction to specific foods as well. You know about the nutrients and vitamins in the foods you eat. And you have some idea about how best to use your ego to keep you on a healthy diet.

This still leaves a great deal to be discussed about food and nutrition—more than can be covered in this book—so I hope you will continue to read about foods and talk about them with your family and friends. In the meantime, it might make good sense to consider some specific foods and food items in terms of how they should (or shouldn't) fit into your diet plans.

In this chapter, we'll take a brief look at some foods that might seem to be good for you, but are really bad for you. And we'll look at some foods that might appear to be bad for you, but are actually good for you. Confused? Don't be. The point is simply this: there are lots of foods with misleading names, or which have a history of misinformation applied to them. Knowing about some of them will help you keep on the lookout for the others.

What's in a name?

You must be careful not to be taken in by a new name stuck on an old familiar product. Nor should you allow yourself to be fooled into eating something whose name implies it might be healthy but which has ingredients you know are bad for you. The most extreme example of this may seem foolish indeed, but I have had adults ask me about it in earnest: we know that baked foods are more healthy than fried foods, but just because the word "baked" appears in Baked Alaska doesn't mean you should run right out and have it every night. And calling greasy French fries by their French name *pommes de terre frites* or *pommes frites* doesn't alter the fact that their oil content is bad for you.

A French fry isn't a vegetable

Potatoes are good for you, but French fries are bad. When I said this in front of a classroom full of schoolchildren, I was answered with a chorus of "But a French fry *is* a potato!" from various little voices all over the room. And I suppose they're right. Yet once the method of preparation is understood, it seems almost beside the point.

Every French fry begins as part of a potato. At this point, it is still very good for you. Potatoes are great. They contain many nutrients, are high in fiber, high in vitamins B and C, and are quite low in calories.

Low in calories? The potato? Right. One reason you have a misperception of the potato being a high-calorie food is the toppings traditionally associated with baked potatoes. You see, the baked potato itself is very good for you. It's the mounds of butter and glaciers of sour cream that make the calorie count go through the roof.

Getting back to the French fry: when the good, healthy potato is sliced up into strips, it is still good for you. Right up until these strips are submerged in a vat of boiling oil they are still good for you. But with the soaking in oil and the boiling hot temperature, all the nutrients and vitamins in the world would be helpless. The onslaught of grease in the average serving of fries would lubricate your car for a week.

If, after that, you still think eating fries is healthy, then you're well on the road toward obesity and heart trouble.

There's milk in a milk shake, isn't there?

Sure, and there's oxygen in car exhaust, too.

Okay, it's unfair to equate the two. Still, you should recognize that drinking a glass of milk is one thing, while having a milk shake is something else again—a less healthy thing. The amount of calcium in each may be approximately the same, but that's about the only similarity. The shake is fattening; milk isn't. The shake has a lot of sugar; milk doesn't. The shake contains artificial colorings and artificial flavorings; milk doesn't.

While you know enough to have something from the dairy food group every day, you should also realize that ice cream, floats, and shakes don't count the way the more healthy foods do—healthy foods like cheese, milk, yogurt, cottage cheese, and so on.

Don't get cheesy

The white cheeses like Swiss, Monterey jack, and Muenster are the best for you because they contain less oil than other cheeses. The light yellow cheeses like gouda and edam are a bit more oily, but these are still better than the yellow cheeses like cheddar and colby. Don't misunderstand—cheese is good for you, but you should not have yellow cheese exclusively.

Whenever possible, try to choose pasteurized cheese rather than processed cheese. The processing removes much of the value of the dairy products used in making cheese. It is not necessarily a matter of taste, although I believe nothing beats the creamy smooth taste of a pasteurized white cheese.

Light beer is still beer

It's hard to avoid hearing and seeing commercials for light beer. They all always make a point about their brand having "fewer calories than regular beer," or something very similar. Only one tells you in large type just how many calories their light beer contains, but the lowest one on the market at present has 70 calories, with other light beers ranging up over 100 calories per bottle or can. All in all, a hefty amount of calories for twelve ounces of water and alcohol. Especially when you consider that 12 ounces of water contains 0 calories.

Besides, light beer is still beer. It can still get you tipsy or drunk, and it still leaves you feeling thirsty so that you're tempted to have more of it. The same can be said of the new low-alcohol beer.

Just because "light" or "low-alcohol" is in the name or on the bottle label, don't think it's a low-calorie, healthy experience.

Candied fruit is more candy than fruit

I've heard adults actually say they were having their fruit for the day when purchasing a box of candied cherries. If they had said it with even a hint of a smile, I'd be ready to believe they were kidding. But no.

Perhaps no one you know is that ignorant, yet it is worthwhile repeating that candied fruit ain't healthy. Even dried fruit, which contains only the natural sugar of the fruit itself, is only good for you in moderation. When purchasing anything other than fresh produce, read the list of ingredients carefully to avoid products with added sugar.

It should be obvious that fresh fruit that is smothered in sweets just isn't the same as having an unadulterated piece of fruit. Caramel apples do indeed contain fresh apples, (perhaps—you don't know when they were covered with caramel), and strawberries dipped in chocolate or powdered sugar are still real strawberries. Yet common sense should tell you something isn't quite right about them. If you want to indulge in such things as a special treat, these are far better than a chocolate dessert without the fruit, but they should not become part of your eating habits.

Make sure things are really popping

If you go to the circus, the ball park, or a movie theater, you can order something to eat which is called popcorn. I suppose there is no legal way to prevent the proprietors of these establishments from using the term popcorn (or, as some of the more unscrupulous ones put it, "fresh popcorn") but it isn't real popcorn as far as I'm concerned.

Real popped corn starts off with actual kernels of corn, and these tiny seeds are heated to popping goodness right before you eat them. Waiting for several hours or longer ruins the whole point of having popcorn. The corn goes stale and loses both flavor and freshness. Reheating it may disguise the fact that it's old—and this is exactly what happens at most places selling "popcorn" these days.

If you've ever been behind the scenes at a movie theater or concession stand, you've seen the same strange sight I once gaped at in amazement: polyethylene bags stuffed with already popped corn. One theater I saw had twenty-eight bags of it lining the back wall of a janitor's service closet.

Think about it: by having a large supply of pre-popped popcorn, the theater doesn't have to train employees to operate a popper. Nor does it have to spend money for the power to run the popper. But it also means that the popcorn you eat may be weeks or months old. That's an insult to your taste buds as well as to your stomach.

Don't settle for old, stale pre-popped corn. If you don't see and hear the kernels popping and gently exploding inside an actual corn popping machine, don't buy the stuff.

If you can find good, fresh popcorn—or if you make it yourself—then it's a good snack food when used in moderation. Popcorn provides roughage, the coarse, bulky substance that helps cleanse your digestive system. Without butter or salt, it's low in calories, too (and that's the only way you should eat it).

Don't add injury to insult

If you eat stale popcorn in a theater, that's an insult. If you have the imitation butter slopped all over it, that's a potential injury. While the proprietors of the concession stands may call it melted butter (which is already bad enough for the popcorn), it really isn't natural butter. Nor is it margarine. It's not much of anything except some chemicals.

You see, it's too much trouble to keep real butter on hand, so a scientifically designed mixture of gelatinous liquid and preservatives is substituted. This stuff can also remain on the shelf for a long time. And usually does. You'd gag if this gunk were spread across your breakfast toast or biscuits, so why settle for it on your popcorn?

The egg and you

Eggs are good protein, but they are high in cholesterol. If you have your eggs fried, you're adding butter or oil that you don't need. Scrambled eggs are better for you, and poached are better still. Best of all are boiled eggs, hard- or soft-boiled.

Sometimes it is possible to go too far with good foods as well as bad. For example, my father likes eggs. A lot. He would have three or four of them every morning if my mother didn't watch out for him. The high level of cholesterol could have a bad effect on his blood pressure, so my mom limits him to a plate of eggs every other morning.

It isn't just high or low blood pressure that may cause a problem with foods that are high in cholesterol. Check with your doctor if you think you might have trouble with cholesterol. Otherwise, don't overdo a good thing like eggs.

Other forms of protein

Meat, fish, and poultry are good sources of protein, yet, as we saw with steak and hamburger, some meats are not good for you. Veal is a good source of protein and is not a fatty meat, but having veal in a French restaurant may be a mistake. It will probably come to you smothered in a sauce that's rich enough to support several emerging nations for a year. French cooking can be a treat, but you should be very careful not to eat full portions, especially if you're not used to it.

Shrimp, like most seafood, is a good source of protein. And, like most fish and shellfish, it is better for you than many meats. This does not justify having a platter of fried shrimp. The deep frying can undo all the good of the protein. And frying practically ruins the whole point of having the shrimp fresh.

Duck is a good source of protein, yet most duck recipes bring out the greasiness of the duck rather than helping remove the grease. And if you order duck in a French restaurant, you're really looking for trouble. It will taste absolutely marvelous, but you may regret having had so much richness at one sitting.

What about a meal of vegetables?

Fine, if you have some protein, dairy foods, and grains at other meals during the day. Very often, vegetables and rice are served together, which combines grain with the fresh veggies.

There can be problems with a type of food that many people associate with vegetables: Chinese food. The trouble is that most American Chinese restaurants serve so many greasy, deep-fried or pan-fried appetizers along with the other food. Added to this is the fact that the rice is almost always fried and often practically dripping with oil. On top of all that is the problem of too much monosodium glutamate. Sodium in any form is to be used only in moderation. You don't have to avoid Chinese food, just be careful about overdoing it.

A potato chip isn't a vegetable

Everything that was said about French fries applies to potato chips (and corn chips, and tortilla chips, and so forth). But the bad news doesn't stop with the oil, because most makers of chips pour on a ton and a half of salt. A little salt in your diet is okay . . . about the amount on three potato chips, say. If you "can't eat just one," can you stop after three?

Cranberry sauce is for turkeys

Sure, it tastes good. And yes, the word "berry" is clearly a part of the name of this food. But cranberry sauce has lots of sugar added to it. Apparently, unadulterated cranberries do not taste very good. I say "apparently" because I've never seen a cranberry. I've seen the juice (which is very good, despite the added sugar). And I've seen the sauce. And that's it.

Cranberry sauce goes very well with turkey, especially turkey that isn't cooked to perfection (the sauce helps disguise the taste of the turkey). Just be aware that you're adding a lot of sugar to your system when you plunk a glob of cranberry sauce on your plate. Only a real turkey would eat too much of it.

The peanut butter conspiracy

There must be some sort of nefarious plot afoot. Peanut butter, which is a good source of protein and other nutritious items, is almost always associated with jams, jellies, candy bars, cookies, and the like. You see commercials for peanut butter 'n' chocolate this and peanut butter 'n' chocolate that. You see ads for peanut butter crunchie candy bars. You read ads about snack foods using peanut butter as a filling.

Only one brand of peanut butter has a national commercial that stresses the nutritional aspect of peanut butter: Skippy. While there are brands with less oil than Skippy, it is a good product that is healthy, nutritious, and delicious.

Certainly you should be careful not to overeat peanut butter, but you might want to keep some around the house for a quick pick-me-up instead of a full-blown meal. If you try one of the so-called old-fashioned brands—in which the oil separates in the jar—you can drain off the extra oil. Open the jar, pour off any oil floating on top, put a folded paper towel across the mouth of the jar, force the twist-top lid back on, and let the whole jar stand upside down on a couple of other paper towels. Leave it for an hour or two.

Whatever brand you buy, you might want to try a peanut butter shake for breakfast. Cut a banana into thin strips and leave in the freezer overnight. Next morning, put the banana strips into a blender with a cup of milk, a half cup of peanut butter, and five large ice cubes. Blend and add honey or cinnamon to taste.

Or try adding some peanut butter to a light syrup in a saucepan. Melt and mix, then serve over pancakes. (Remember, moderation is best when dealing with a sugary substance like syrup.)

A different kind of pie

There is a type of pie which, when eaten in moderate portions, can provide you with nutrients from at least three of the four basic food groups. In fact, depending on the style of pie ordered, you might get something from all four food groups.

This particular pie can be a whole meal in itself. By now, you've probably guessed the kind of pie I'm talking about: pizza pie.

Okay, okay, so I misled you a bit. Hardly anybody calls it pizza pie anymore, but that is the original and proper name.

Pizza is good food. When it's prepared properly, the oil level isn't too high (beware of those places serving an oily product; they're trying to cover up something) and the dough isn't too rich (watch out for places serving chewy dough; it's overly rich without adding to the taste of the pizza). The reasons people have reservations about pizza have more to do with the way they eat it than with the product itself.

Pizza is finger food. As such, it's fun to eat. The good time, party atmosphere can induce some of us to eat faster than we should, and eating faster usually leads to eating more than necessary. Then, too, the pizza is a bit hot in your hands, so you have a natural tendency to take a hurried chomp out of the slice you're holding instead of a more dignified bite or dainty nibble.

Having only one or two slices of pizza, no matter how loaded with ingredients, never seems like an entire meal, so people keep eating beyond their normal stopping point. In addition, pizza just seems to go with beer, so that's another reason people associate pizza with a high-calorie meal—they pig out by having too many slices of the pizza, then they down too many pitchers of brew. No wonder the word "pizza" can connote a stuffed, bloated feeling.

If this is how you treat pizza, it simply will not work as part of The Ego Diet. But if you consider exactly what goes into a pizza, you may find that you've discovered a great way to get good food into your body while enjoying a taste treat.

Every good pizza starts with fresh dough for the crust. While I have not seen a commercially available whole wheat crust pizza, the grain in a regular pizza crust is still good for you. After tomato sauce (which should be made from fresh tomatoes) is spread on the dough, cheese is sprinkled, grated, or layered on top. Good pizza restaurants use 100 percent real cheese, a dairy product that also provides protein. You can get more protein if you decide to order meat toppings. You do have to be careful to watch out for the fatty meats like ground beef and some salamis, but the better pizza parlors have good pepperoni (still on the fatty side of things, but acceptable in small quantities). You can stick to the vegetable toppings, however, and really make your pizza healthy.

Good pizza makers use fresh mushrooms, fresh green (bell) pepper, and fresh tomatoes, and all of these make for a delicious and nutritious pizza. Some places serve a pizza with ham and pineapple, so you can even get fruit with your pizza.

Remember, each slice of pizza is like holding a couple of pieces of toast, an order of vegetables, the cheese from a grilled cheese sandwich, plus whatever meats you have selected. If you keep in mind that you're holding essentially a whole plate of food in your hand, you won't eat as much at one sitting. (Besides, leftover pizza is good cold right out of the refrigerator for lunch the next day.)

Your choice

Whenever you make a decision about eating, you're controlling your diet. You can give in to the whim of the moment, or you can remain in charge of the situation. You can succumb to the dictates of your taste buds, or you can stay steadfast in your desire to perfect your body.

You don't have to fight the whole war when these decision points are reached. Just take them one at a time. Just win this current battle. That's all.

And please—give your body a break; stick to the good foods whenever you can.

20

Some Diet Methods To Avoid

EVERY diet plan involves some time and effort to make it successful. Usually, the more time and the more effort, the more successful the diet plan.

The Ego Diet takes work, although the many side benefits may compensate somewhat for the strain. And the time needed for The Ego Diet is deliberately extended over the longest period of time humanly possible: the rest of your life. The fact that it offers such a good and sensible balance of food, nutrition, and diet makes The Ego Diet essential in your life. And as for the effort required for the diet plan to work, since The Ego Diet makes use of a power source located inside you, there is less sweat with this plan than with most others.

But what about a "no effort" diet?

Ah, that has been the dream of every potentially lazy person in the world (that is to say, all of us) since the word overweight was first used. "Wouldn't it be nice if you could eat as much as you want and never gain any weight?" You've heard overweight people say this. You may have said it, too. Well, forget it. That kind of wishful thinking ignores your psychological need for feelings of security (which you get partially through food). It disavows your association of pleasure with taste. It overlooks the fact that raising your blood-sugar level (which is accomplished by eating) brings about a very real physical boost. And it is blind to the impossibility of not gaining weight if you take in more calories than you burn.

Still, the dream of a "no work" diet plan lives inside us. And this makes us fair game for the come-ons of the double-faced, pettifogging glad-handers who are out to cheat and swindle their way to a fat bank account. Many a charlatan has sold a bill of goods to many a sucker by the simple method of calling snake oil a "miracle diet" that promises quick, permanent weight loss without the bother of such sticky details as time or effort. Only money is required.

"Step right up, folks," runs the spiel, "and let me show you the eighth wonder of the world, the first wonder of the universe: a way to lose weight in your sleep!" (Or "while lying down!" Or "by taking this little pill!" Or . . . but you get the picture.)

Let's get something straight. There are no miracle diets. You want to lose weight? Fine—*you* lose the weight. You are in control. Not a pill or a machine, you.

Yes, I know that you've heard and read about people losing large numbers of pounds in amazingly short periods of time. And some people do, indeed, lose weight in this manner. Very few people, actually, but there are some folks who will swear to having permanently lost pounds in some weird way. What they don't tell you are the side effects or that in order to maintain their health they had to abandon the "miracle" method and adopt a traditional diet plan.

In this chapter I'm going to tell you the stories behind the so-called super diets. Before dealing with each one individually, I want to let you know about something many of them have in common. The ads for these diets often feature some variation of the phrase, "approved by doctors." Sounds impressive, doesn't it? But all it means is that physicians and attorneys specializing in medical law could find no legal reason why the sale of the diet method in question should be prevented. It in no way implies an endorsement or even a recommendation. Many doctors don't even wish to condone these methods, but if the snake oil doesn't actually harm people, it can go on being sold.

The diet connection

Diet pills. They're truly a drug on the market, and they sell like crazy. You can get them over the counter at supermarkets, and you can get the stronger stuff at pharmacies. They're a multimillion dollar industry—more than fourteen million individual prescriptions are written each year in this country alone.

The overwhelming majority of the prescription drugs for people attempting to diet are amphetamines, the so-called diet pills you hear people talk about. There are a great many problems and side effects caused by the use of these drugs, as you'll see.

Amphetamines are prescribed for some medical purposes other than weight control. For example, they are used to treat some forms of minor brain dysfunction. They are also prescribed to treat narcolepsy (an illness characterized by attacks of very deep sleep—which is why some of the lighter doses of amphetamines are used in the "stay awake" pills people sometimes use).

In the treatment of those other medical problems, it was noted that one of the side effects of the drug was the suppression of appetite. Pharmaceutical manufacturers developed pills that acted more as an appetite killer than as a medication for mental disorders (or so they said), and the diet pill craze was on. Unfortunately, the taking of diet pills also suppresses treatment of the problem of overeating. When the taking of pills is stopped—which must happen sooner or later—the problem remains and the patient gains weight once more.

Meanwhile, use of amphetamines increases blood pressure and heart rate, brings on attacks of acute anxiety, and may even lead to minor brain damage and psychotic episodes. Long-term use of amphetamines has produced cases of brain hemorrhage (the bursting of blood vessels in the brain). The street name for amphetamines is speed. The street talk warning about it is "speed kills." No jive.

It is also possible to become addicted to amphetamines. A physical and psychological dependence on drugs is not pretty. While Hollywood has made the addict who craves his or her next fix somewhat of a cliché, the ugly reality of a once-rational human being scrounging for stolen or illicitly produced drugs just to feed a habit is not to be ignored. Every one of the well-meaning, primarily middle-to-upper-class people who have become addicted to diet pills started out thinking it couldn't happen to them.

After using any drug for a short period of time, your body begins to adapt to the effects of the drug. This leads to the desire for more drugs—either an increased dosage or the same dosage repeated more often. This tolerance level buildup is exactly the same as the tolerance level buildup experienced by users of alcohol (see Chapter 17).

Using drugs indiscriminately will break down your will power. Prisoners captured in the Korean War were given high and repeated dosages of drugs in order to make them more compliant. Under this attack from within their own bodies, many soldiers more readily gave information to their captors, signed false confessions, and so forth. Obviously, any breakdown of will power is counter to the goals of The Ego Diet, quite apart from the fact that it isn't healthy.

You sometimes hear the excuse that diet pills are necessary for an individual because of a hormone problem or a thyroid condition. Either one of these explanations may be true, but it isn't likely. In only about 2 percent of the recorded cases of overweight people seeking medical help did a hormonal imbalance or thyroid hyperactivity (or thyroid misfunction) show up. In other words, the odds are that anyone who is overweight and using diet pills doesn't need to do so. The hormone and thyroid stories are just that—stories. They're simply a way to justify taking the lazy way out. People who do this are taking a large risk for their laziness.

One other side effect of amphetamines needs mentioning. Although it is relatively minor when compared to dependence (a drug habit) and death, it has often produced more fear among potential users than anything else. It is bad breath. The use of amphetamines can cause a foul mouth odor because of the body's chemical reactions to the drug.

If fear of bad breath is what it takes to keep you away from diet pills, so be it. I would have been willing to bet on death as the primary dissuader, but then that would have been a logical reaction, and there is nothing logical about drug use.

The bathroom drug

To prevent the problems caused by amphetamines, some physicians have chosen to prescribe diuretic drugs for their patients who wish to lose weight without using their will power. A diuretic is a drug that forces the body to eliminate water, or pass water. You'll spend a fair amount of time going to and fro between the bathrooms at home or office if you use diuretics.

This is a phony way to lose weight, because the body, with its built-in regulatory system, will retain water from whatever is eaten after the diuretic wears off. And as for whatever you eat and drink while the drug is in your body, since the diuretic is forcing an unnatural and speeded-up regimen of elimination, you are missing out on the nutrients that would have been absorbed into your system had the food and drink only been allowed to remain inside you for a normal and proper length of time. (Many foods contain quite a bit of water, so the vitamins and minerals in many "solid" foods are washed away with the water if diuretics are used.)

It is certainly true that a diuretic will enable you to take off several pounds in a short space of time. Yet the use of this kind of drug also virtually guarantees that you'll regain the pounds when a normal intake of food and drink is resumed after the use of the drug is stopped.

At this point, the truly lazy person thinks, "Well, I'll just keep on taking the diuretic so I'll never have to diet again." There are two things wrong with this line of thinking. First, you would be shortchanging your body in terms of vital nutrients. Second, and more important, you'd soon experience kidney malfunctions. And this could quickly become very serious, because the kidneys perform a crucial function in your elimination of waste materials from your body. Unlike a Gila monster, which retains some of its own waste matter to use as a poison, humans die if waste isn't removed from their bodies.

Liquid protein diets

No, this is not the opposite of diuretics. A liquid protein diet requires you to mix powdered protein with water (or some other liquid) or to use a premixed solution as your only food source for a certain period of time. The calorie intake on such a diet may be as low as 330 calories a day. Advertisements and paid testimonials for such diets proclaim astonishing weight losses for people using these liquids.

But then again, perhaps the weight losses they shout about are not so astonishing when you consider how drastic a diet they offer. The chief of the nutrition and metabolism laboratory of New England Deaconess Hospital, Dr. George Blackburn, speaking for this nation's health and nutrition experts, said that they agreed no diet of less than 800 calories a day be attempted without medical supervision. That figure is 800 daily calories—yet some of the liquid protein diets have you taking less than half that amount.

People have died from liquid protein diets. The people didn't starve to death—there wasn't time for that—most became ill from their weakened condition and were unable to fight off disease.

One advertisement for one of the more famous liquid protein diet plans put it this way:

> If you were starving on a desert island you would not lose body fat faster . . .

I suppose the only other logical comparison one could make between a drastic diet plan and a horrible crisis situation would be a concentration camp. This whole line of reasoning I find distasteful in the extreme, yet this is how they choose to advertise their wares.

Much discussion of liquid protein diets has centered on the type of protein used in the preparation of the formula. It is claimed that the deaths associated with the craze of liquid protein diets resulted more from the low-quality protein than from the incredibly low number of calories in the daily plan. The newer liquid protein mixes, it is further claimed, use a higher grade of protein derived from milk. Even if better protein is being used and though I certainly approve of using the highest form of protein available, I think these diet plans can be dangerous. Beware of any diet plan that limits you to less than 800 calories a day. Hurting your body is bad enough; risking death is ridiculous.

The disgorge dilemma

Far from being the title of another Robert Ludlum book, the disgorge dilemma is the problem faced by the person who tries to reduce or maintain weight by vomiting.

I'm sorry to have to bring this disgusting practice to your attention, but it is a diet method that some people believe is worth considering. If this is something you know you will never consider, and you wish to avoid reading about it, please skip to the next section.

The practice of deliberately disgorging food began in ancient times during a period marked by much conspicuous consumption by the aristocracy. Feasts were held during which it became fashionable to eat as much as possible in the space of a day or more. In order to keep eating without bursting, habitués of these events would induce vomiting to empty the contents of their stomachs at periodic intervals.

For some strange reason, this revolting habit has become a fascinating diet plan for the supposedly more enlightened citizens of the modern world. There are quite a few drawbacks to this weird system of unnatural elimination.

First, it's dangerous in the immediate physical sense. Your body goes into a convulsion when you force your fingers down your throat. It is an extremely violent reaction, and it is meant to take place only when your body absolutely must rid itself of a foreign substance like tainted food. The rush of half-digested food up your throat is virtually uncontrollable. People who are otherwise quite healthy have choked to death from their own vomit because their air passages became accidently clogged. I once had difficulty disgorging food after having consumed contaminated meat. I went into a state of hyperventilation, with my arms and legs turning both numb and rigid.

Second, it is psychologically dangerous. Repeated use of this method of reducing food intake could cause you to associate the act of eating with the act of vomiting. If you make this association voluntarily as part of your ego behavior control, you may be able to manage your eating habits both during and after relying on this technique (see Chapter 22). But if you cannot help recalling the act of vomiting when you even think of food—because the physical and emotional sense-memory is too strong—then you could be in a bad state. You might be faced with the problem of anorexia.

Third, it is very bad for you from the standpoint of nutrition. By inducing a physical reaction that removes food from your stomach, you prevent your body from digesting the food. This means you are not allowing the nutrients to be extracted from the food and utilized by your body. You could actually suffer from vitamin deficiency while using this method, no matter how much good, healthy food you eat.

Fourth, this activity can damage your throat and nasal passages. The acids that are removed from your stomach along with the food cause a burning sensation. It is a normal reaction to the harsh, biting nature of these strong liquids. While this damage is uncommon unless repeated doses are allowed to attack your nose and throat, it is a danger that can so easily be avoided it seems silly to run even the slight risk.

Fifth, you put your body through muscle spasms that are debilitating. One person using this method told me she was glad she was "getting some more exercise" when she was down on her knees hugging the toilet bowl. Although I laughed sardonically at the time, I knew she was getting the wrong type of exercise. If you were able to notice (or care) the last time you experienced it, your abdomen, upper and lower back, neck, and shoulders were all tensing and flexing in a violent manner. This is hardly a healthy form of exercise. Strained muscles and/or torn ligaments can be the result.

Sixth, it is messy.

Seventh, it is something you don't want your partner, spouse, relatives, or friends to see or know about unless you are truly ill. Otherwise, it is like crying wolf. Someday you might have the misfortune to be struck by food poisoning and need medical help—if you have a history of going through this activity on a stupid whim, you might not get the help you need when it really counts.

This is a very unwise solution to the problem of overeating. It is a coward's way out and a fool's way to flirt with danger. Don't do it.

All wrapped up

Body wrapping is a relatively new weight-loss stratagem, yet it is somewhat similar to the old steamroom/sweatbox reducing method. Various types of wrapping material are utilized by different wrapping systems, but the process is pretty much the same wherever you go.

Essentially, your body is put into a cocoon of nonporous fabric or plastic. Nonporous literally means "no pores," so the effect is like wearing a plastic bag—your body can't breathe because no air enters or leaves the material.

Have you ever worn a very cheap pair of shoes, ones made from plastic or imitation leather? What happens when you wear shoes like this? Your feet sweat because they cannot get air. If you didn't have socks to soak up some of the perspiration (and to provide some small distance for air space between your skin and the shoe), your feet would very nearly puff up and explode from being parboiled.

As you might guess, the proprietors of body-wrapping parlors are able to claim fabulous amounts of weight loss in very short periods of time for their vict—— um, customers. This is because the wrapping forces the water from the body. Also as you might guess, this water loss is as phony as a weight loss from using diuretics.

Most body-wrapping places are probably clean, but there is a real problem with bacteria if the owners or managers do not enforce high standards of cleanliness. While the wrapping method is generally worthless in the long run, you can obtain a quick weight loss from it if necessary—provided you find a clean, well-run establishment. If you even suspect the place isn't as clean as it should be, get out of there fast.

"Look into my eyes . . ."

With the showing of such Hollywood semiclassics as *Svengali, Black Magic, Fear in the Night* and its remake *Nightmare,* the late-night television viewing public gains interest in hypnosis. There are, of course, many more examples of hypnosis on screen. *On A Clear Day You Can See Forever* and *Freud* come immediately to mind, as well as the Pat Collins appearance in *Divorce American Style.* The uses of hypnosis in television episodes are too numerous to mention.

In film after film and TV show after TV show, some character is shown performing some act that defies logic or sensibility—at least the sensibility of the particular character being portrayed at the time. In *Fear in the Night* and *Nightmare,* for example, the hero is hypnotized into becoming a murderer. In *Whirlpool,* Jose Ferrer hypnotizes himself into leaving his hospital bed and committing a murder.

Because of this, people have come to believe that hypnotism can help them solve their problems. The logic seems to be that if hypnotism is powerful enough to make people commit murder it will also be powerful enough to work on their "impossible" bad habits. Alcoholics try hypnosis to keep them away from booze. Sports figures try it to improve their game. People in business use it to help them overcome a fear of public speaking. Overweight people try it to see if it will help them stop overeating.

With all this hypnotic activity, are there any risks, particularly with regard to the hypnotic state itself?

In John Frankenheimer's film version of Richard Condon's *The Manchurian Candidate,* one of the physicians in an early scene tells the other characters that it is a mistake to believe people under hypnosis won't do anything that they wouldn't ordinarily do. Whereupon he orders one of the hypnotized subjects in the room to shoot one of his Army buddies. Which he does. Of course, the subjects were also under the influence of drugs. Still, it is worth considering that phrase "wouldn't ordinarily do." Naturally, none of us goes around committing murder "ordinarily." Yet the hypnotic state itself is out of the ordinary, so there may be room for doubt as to the safety of being given a posthypnotic suggestion.

Furthermore, just what unusual behavior lies under the otherwise ordinary surface of each of us? Isn't it possible that many hopes, hates, and desires are never fully expressed because of a natural or learned inhibition or a fear of getting caught? Could not the hypnotic state then be the excuse needed for the expression of these feelings and impulses?

Right about now, the ethical, licensed psychiatrists and therapists who use hypnosis only in a helping, healthy manner are getting ready to aim a blast of negative reaction in the direction of this book.

But they shouldn't be angry with me. They should direct their wrath at those charlatans and clowns who promise miracle cures through hypnosis, or who reduce hypnosis to the level of a party game. These are the people who cause me to consider the possible ill use of hypnosis.

Now, to partially counteract the above reservations, I would like to say that hypnosis *may* be an acceptable way for some individuals to begin modifying their diet plans and their mind-set concerning food and eating. You will have to discuss this with your doctor, and possibly a psychiatrist.

There are hypnosis experts who agree that all hypnosis is in reality a form of self-hypnosis. Many subjects of hypnosis state that they were aware of the "act" of the person performing the hypnotic "spell." They still wanted to go along with the hypnotist. As one man at a party put it, "You know the guy is taking you somewhere and you just have to want to go along with him." To which I replied, "It sounds a lot like buying a used car."

If all hypnosis involves a voluntary action on the part of the participant, then the rest is merely a surrendering of will power to the hypnotist. Yet this does not explain the demonstrations of people going rigid when on stage in a hypnosis performance.

So it may be that the effect differs from person to person. Which way would it be with you? Would you "go along" with the hypnotist, or would you completely surrender your soul? Would you, as so many people believe, be perfectly safe because you wouldn't do anything wrong? Or would you commit some act you wouldn't be capable of performing under normal circumstances?

It is true that many people have been aided by hypnosis, so my raising your level of fear may not be entirely fair. Still, I feel that any weight-control help you get from a hypnotist is likely to be of value only in the short run. Carried out over a long period of time, it represents a dangerous reliance on another person who is in business, with you as the client. Only a psychiatrist should perform hypnosis, in my opinion.

On the other hand, if you are able to learn to reinforce your own posthypnotic suggestions, then you would be merely substituting another method for The Ego Diet methods. Or perhaps you would be augmenting one method with another. Either way, if this can be accomplished, more power to you. I do feel, however, that anyone strong enough to learn true self-hypnosis is strong enough to rely on his or her own ego.

There is a monetary consideration here. If you were to attempt to obtain the services of a hypnotist each time the posthypnotic suggestion wore off, you would be paying a lot of money for something you can do for yourself.

Going under the knife

When a person has eaten his or her way up to twice normal size, it may well be that drastic measures are in order. In many cases of extreme obesity, surgery is attempted as a last resort attack on the problem of overeating.

When this solution was first developed, it was an intestinal bypass operation that limited the amount of food that could be held in the intestine, and with less food held there, less could be digested. Consequently, the patient was forced to lose weight.

This particular surgical procedure had many dangerous side effects. As a result, the practice has been abandoned in favor of a new technique. Now, the operation takes place farther up the gastrointestinal tract, essentially reducing the volume of the stomach.

Operating on the stomach to make it smaller has risks of its own. There is, first of all, always a risk in any form of surgery involving general anesthesia (the act of "putting you under" or using drugs to make you black out). This risk is only increased by being overweight to start with. Second, and more important (also more likely), is the problem of infection at the point of the surgery. Another problem is the body's rejection of the "tied-off" tummy. A fourth problem is one of vomiting, which is fairly common, especially if the patient does not adequately cut back on food intake. And finally, since this is a relatively new procedure, other unknown complications may emerge.

Only if the above-mentioned difficulties are overcome will this radical method of weight control be successful. Because it is such an extreme, unusual, and scary procedure, physicians will not consider it for anyone who isn't at least 100 pounds overweight.

The electric diet

Think about walking into a small private clinic, removing your clothing, and lying down on a table. Someone attaches electrodes to your body and then throws a switch, sending countless electric shocks through your flesh. Sound like fun? How about if it took place in a storefront office that had been converted from an old hardware store or tarot card reading parlor? (The latter descriptions seem to suit the kinds of places indulging in this activity.)

This is one of the latest "no work" reducing plans. The electric shocks (or, in some cases, some sort of ultrasonic shocks) cause your muscles to contract over and over again very rapidly. This forces you to move even while you are lying down.

While it seems as if this method of weight reduction couldn't miss (for those souls who dig this kind of punishment), apparently the procedure lulls the participant into a false sense of security regarding food and exercise. What happens is that even less attention is paid to proper diet. This may lead to the person increasing the visits to the shock parlor, which is not only expensive, it can prove debilitating in the long run.

Killer exercise plans

I've known people who have finished a good-sized meal and headed outside for "some exercise to work off the pounds of food." Do not exercise immediately after eating. Taking a leisurely stroll is fine, but trying to race around the tennis court is suicide (or it could be, anyway).

By the same token, devising an exercise plan that works your body to the point of exhaustion is foolish and unnecessary. If you are being supervised by a physical therapist or trainer, then you can follow orders and assume that the pain you're enduring has some point. Otherwise, a killer exercise plan can become a real killer.

21

Eating For Fuel Versus Eating For Taste

WE have already seen why you get hungry: your blood sugar drops. But why do you eat? In particular, why do you eat when you're not hungry?

You see a cupcake in a sweet-shop window, and what happens? If you are letting your taste buds control your behavior, you think about going into the shop and buying the cupcake. Or three. If you've learned to harness the power of your ego, you immediately get a warning sign flashed to your brain that says "danger." You know that the taste is a transitory pleasure but the sugar has an effect that can last a long time as added fat on your body.

Those people who consume food primarily for taste are certainly standouts. They stand out in the belly, in the hips, in the thighs, in the bottom, and in a dozen other places.

You don't want to be like these people. You are different in dozens of other ways, so you should be different in your approach to food.

It begins in your head

Your brain controls part of your taste reaction. If you want to become healthy, you'll begin to question the worth of the stuff you put into your mouth. That's an important step toward losing weight now and maintaining your ideal weight in the future.

You may be saying to yourself, "I don't want to go on a health-food diet." You don't have to become a health-food junkie, just try to avoid even approaching the problems of a junk-food junkie.

Just ask yourself . . .

"Do I want to taste this food, or do I need it in my stomach for fuel?"

That one question alone will go a long way toward helping you control your diet. It might also help to compare what you're considering eating with something else that is also available. When someone in your office brings in doughnuts, your taste buds might make you begin salivating for the taste of sugar and dough. Don't be ashamed of it—the same thing happens to me. Just take a second to ask yourself if you feel the same way about having an orange or apple. If not, perhaps you aren't really hungry. In which case, skip the doughnuts. If you do feel like eating the fruit, great—eat the fruit. You'll enjoy the natural fruit sugar and be helping the rest of your body at the same time.

Cravings

Sometimes your body is trying to tell you something. Other times, the craving you feel for sugar or fat is purely taste oriented. In this country, we grow up with the instant gratification from a new taste sensation every day. A hundred flavors of ice cream. Cookies. Doughnuts. Candy bars galore. And I haven't even begun listing the deep-fried foods.

We indulge in these taste sensations to the exclusion of the natural taste sensations available all around us. Why this should be so is something philosophers have been worrying about ever since hedonistic societies first began placing a greater value on the fadish elements of the world than on the solid virtues. I believe that the taste cravings we all experience are a symptom of weakness that should be tamed. You know you've conquered your problem when you begin salivating at the thought of whole wheat bread or bran muffins rather than a glazed piece of coffee cake.

The change can happen suddenly

If you are like me, you think you'll never lose your desire for sugar or fat. But it can happen. It happened to me. Sure, I still have a doughnut every now and then. But I stop after the first one (or after the first half), whereas before The Ego Diet I would gladly have three or four of them.

After a few months of deliberately searching out the good foods, I suddenly began looking forward to the taste of broccoli, something I had loathed in the past. I was quite surprised, but that day I went out to lunch at a Thai restaurant and ordered chicken and broccoli, one of their specialties. It was incredibly delicious. The subtle blend of tastes was something I had never before been able to appreciate. My taste buds had become so dulled by the bad foods that I didn't really taste what good food had to offer.

Now I wanted more information about other good and bad foods. What was I currently eating that would get in the way of my appreciating the fruits, vegetables, and grains I knew I should have been eating all along?

I began examining the foods I thought tasted good and asked myself if they provided my body with good, pure fuel. If the answer was "no," then I wanted to learn why. In this manner, I felt I would be able to change the way I reacted to them. There was no way of knowing if my taste buds would change any more than they already had, but one thing was certain: I was going to discover the truth behind the foods that were being marketed to all of us through ads, promotions, and coupons.

Sugar (and hidden sugar)

There are at least twenty-one different kinds or forms of sugar, but a sugar by any other name will taste as sweet. Unfortunately, it will also act on your body the same way.

Until the mid-1970s, most sugar was extracted from sugar cane or beets. Around 1974, a number of factors combined to vastly increase the price of this method of making sugar, and this led to the making of corn sugar, sometimes called corn sweetener or even fructose corn syrup. With the new name, and a growing public awareness of the importance of natural foods, manufacturers began substituting these new names for the word sugar on their ingredients lists (which must, by law, appear on the label of any food product sold in the United States).

But under any of those names, sugar is still sugar. In fact, all the names listed below mean sugar, despite differences in the chemical composition of each product.

Manufactured or Refined Sugars

Sucrose (the white granulated sugar found in most sugarbowls)
Glucose, dextrose (both names refer to the same product)
Lactose (sugar made from milk)
Fructose, levulose
Maltose

Natural Sugars

Maltitol
Mannitol
Xylitol (found in birch trees)
Sorbitol
All of these, except xylitol, are found in fruit.

When reading a product label list of ingredients, you may see any of these names, but they all stand for the same sweet thing.

By mixing these forms of sugar in different ways, other forms of sugar can be made. All the food items listed below—many of which may not normally be thought of as sugar—actually contain up to 98 percent sucrose:

> Honey (fructose, glucose, sucrose, and maltose)
> Corn syrup (fructose and dextrose)
> Brown sugar (white sugar with molasses)
> Kleenraw sugar (white sugar with about 5 percent molasses)
> Light brown sugar
> Surbinado sugar (just a white sugar made with a spinning process)
> Raw sugar (just a made-up name for one of the other sugars—it is against the law to sell raw sugar for consumption in the U.S., because sugar must be refined to remove foreign substances)

All sugars are simple carbohydrates (a chemical compound made up of carbon, hydrogen, and oxygen). By "simple," I mean that the number of molecules forming the product is small. This makes it easy for your body to break it down very fast. A more complex carbohydrate, like a potato or a pear, gives your digestive system more to work with, which is much healthier for you.

The simplest forms of sugar are fructose and glucose and it is these two which, when combined, form the most familiar sugar: sucrose—the kind you put in your coffee at the lunch counter. Even when fructose and glucose are combined to form sucrose, your body can still break it down very rapidly. The so-called sugar rush that you feel after eating cookies or a candy bar on an empty stomach comes about because the glucose gets into your bloodstream in a flash. The higher level of glucose in the blood triggers your pancreas to produce insulin (a hormone that makes it possible for glucose to be used by your body and regulates sugar levels in the blood).

The more sugar-heavy junk food you eat, the more insulin is produced. Your pancreas can, however, be overloaded or overstimulated. If this occurs, too much insulin will be produced, leading to hypoglycemia, a condition caused by too little sugar in the blood. That's correct—eating too much sugar causes the body to produce too much insulin, which takes too much sugar out of your system. It seems backward when you first hear it, but eating too much sugar will bring on an illness characterized by too little sugar.

The typical hypoglycemic reactions are hunger, headache, dizziness, overheating with profuse sweating, severe irritability, depression, anger, and an inability to sleep. As the amount of insulin produced in your body rises, you risk convulsions and unconsciousness.

All of these problems can be avoided by taking your sugar in complex carbohydrates like fruit. (The other complex carbohydrates are vegetables and grains, and while some of them contain some natural sugar, fruit contains the most.) The natural sugar in an apple is combined with fiber, vitamins, and minerals. Sugar in fibrous foods is by far the easiest on your system.

Quite apart from the fiber is the fact that your body was made to digest the natural sugars, not the refined ones. When you eat refined sugar without fiber, you shock your system. The problem is compounded by the large amounts of refined sugar in most sweets. To get the same amount of sugar as in a four-ounce candy bar, you'd have to eat about eight apples.

If all of the above were not enough, there's the major health hazard from eating sweets: cavities. Tooth decay is not as dramatic a reason as hypoglycemia for avoiding sugar, but it is a very real problem. The high sugar content of candies and other goodies is made worse by the fact that many of these foods are quite sticky—the worst type of food for your teeth. To avoid problems of tooth decay, brush after eating. If you can't brush, rinse with water.

There is one bright spot to this section. Contrary to popular belief, too much sugar does not appear to cause diabetes. Although heredity is the principal factor, many people struck by diabetes, especially those over forty, are overweight. While it is true that many overweight people eat a great deal of sugar, not all do. Some people simply eat until their bodies are stuffed, carefully avoiding sugar "because of the calories." They still gain weight, and they still can get diabetes.

Your body does need sugar, but the best way to get it is by eating foods with other nutrients besides natural sugars. If you can train yourself to eat fruit instead of cookies, you'll find that your taste buds will gradually come alive, enabling you to enjoy the smaller amounts of natural sugars in apples, pears, oranges, melons, and the like.

The junk foods that contain a lot of sugar also contain oodles of calories, yet they provide no nutrition. They have what some people call "empty calories." When eating food of this nature, you are truly cheating your body. You are eating for taste instead of for fuel.

250 calories per ounce

No wonder it's called "fat." With 250 calories to the ounce, fat is a heavy load on your plate. And it becomes a heavy load to carry around all day when it attaches itself to your body. By comparison, carbohydrates and protein average around 125 calories per ounce.

Unlike sugars, which come in different forms, fat is just fat. The fat in margarine is the same as the fat in butter . . . is the same as the fat in nuts . . . is the same as the fat in deep-fried foods. While your body needs some fat in your diet, you could probably benefit from consuming one-third less fat daily.

We have already discussed the role cholesterol plays in hurting your body—how it builds up in your arteries—and cholesterol is a fatlike substance that is in saturated fat. Again, while your body needs some cholesterol, most people could profitably cut back.

Eating too much saturated fat causes your cholesterol level to rise alarmingly (not to mention the added pounds you'll be wearing). Foods with a lot of saturated fat include meat, butter, cream, and cheese. You probably eat too much fatty meat and use too much butter (I did before The Ego Diet), but you probably are well within the acceptable limits when it comes to eating cheese. This last assumption seems a pretty safe guess, because we in this country don't make a meal of cheese and bread as some Europeans do. But then again, there are all those wine and cheese parties . . .

"What about unsaturated fats?" someone usually asks. "Aren't they better for you than saturated fats?" Sure, but only because they are a bit easier to digest. If you have a choice between cooking with unsaturated fats like vegetable oil and corn oil or cooking with butter, by all means choose the vegetable-based oil. Just don't think that you can increase the amount of unsaturated fat just because you're cutting back on the saturated stuff.

Eating too much of any kind of fat will, in essence, clog up your fuel lines (your bloodstream). Your arteries must remain free of cholesterol if you expect to keep a smooth-running engine (body).

The U.S. Dietary Guidelines for a low-fat, low-unsaturated fat, and low-cholesterol diet are as follows:

Eat lean meat, poultry, fish, dry beans, peas.
Monitor and moderate your use of eggs, shellfish, and meats
from organs (like liver).
Cut down on your use of butter, margarine, cream, shortening,

and both palm oil and coconut oil (two exceptions to the rule that vegetable oils are unsaturated).

Trim excess fat from meat.

Broil, boil, or bake foods rather than frying them.

Salt of the earth

Do you put salt on your food? Why? I know you don't do it for fuel, because your body gets all the salt it needs from the fairly high sodium levels in meat, fish, poultry, grains, fruits, and vegetables.

So if you're adding salt to your food either while cooking or at the table, you're only doing it for taste.

Like many of us, you have slowly had your taste buds dulled by rushing through poorly prepared meals adulterated with salt and products high in salt. The salt, in its various guises, like some of those listed below, is simply used to give tasteless food a "kick." It is a transitory thing for each meal, but over years of use, you begin to expect it on everything. A friend once told me about someone he knew in the Army who put Tabasco sauce on everything, including his morning eggs. When questioned about this habit, he said, "Where I come from, we like things hot. If I don't put this on my food, I can't taste anything."

Although salt isn't as violent on your tongue as Tabasco, it will attack your taste buds, especially when used too often. Since salt is already in food, and it is in so many things that are added to food, you can really get overloaded with it. Here are some foods notably high in sodium or added salt:

Soy sauce
Steak sauce
Pickled foods (like relish)
Mustard, ketchup
Cured meats
Potato chips, corn chips
Salted nuts, popcorn, and pretzels
Foods with MSG (monosodium glutimate, like most American-style Chinese food)
Hot dogs, sausage
Most processed meats, but not all (read ingredients list on the label before buying: they are listed in order by weight, heaviest first)

Added salt in food is an acquired taste. You can gradually learn to like foods without adding salt. If you cut out added salt for a brief period, you'll find that foods begin to taste good without it. You'll discover that peanuts in the shell taste better than salted peanuts. You can prepare foods with herbs and lemon juice rather than using the lazy cook's additives: onion salt, garlic salt, salty sauces, and other sodium-rich condiments.

You get enough salt in the good foods—anywhere from a third of a teaspoon up to three-quarters of a teaspoon per day—to maintain a proper mixture of fuel in your system. Think about holding a teaspoon nearly full of salt up to your mouth. That's how much salt you're already eating daily. Keep that image in mind whenever you think about adding more salt to your food.

Or think about this: the risk of high blood pressure is the penalty for eating too much salt. And the risks associated with high blood pressure include kidney trouble, heart disease, and stroke. Salt just isn't worth the risk.

A liberal who is conservative

Former Senator George McGovern, when he was chairman of the Senate Select Committee on Nutrition and Human Needs, issued a set of dietary guidelines very similar to those of The Ego Diet. If I had been aware of these guidelines earlier, I might not have developed The Ego Diet, so I'm happy I didn't run across them. Still, it is a shame this information cannot be made more readily available to people.

I can certainly commend Senator McGovern for his committee's work, and I gladly pass on some of its findings.

Since the average American's diet was studied on a massive scale, these conclusions have more, uh, weight than many others. It was found that on the average, our diet is made up of the following:

fat—42 percent
protein—12 percent
carbohydrates—46 percent

It was also found that there is an ideal diet for the average person, and it looks like this:

fat—30 percent
protein—12 percent
carbohydrates—58 percent

The important thing to notice here is that you don't have to cut back on eating in order to have a healthier body and a trimmer figure. Just cut your fat intake by one-third and substitute carbohydrates like vegetables, rice, potatoes, and grains (but remember to go easy on the fatty stuff like butter when you're making or serving these foods!).

It is interesting to note that, with this one recommendation alone, the Senate Committee predicted these very healthy results:

An 80 percent drop in the number of overweight citizens
A 1 percent increase in overall life expectancy
A 25 percent drop in heart disease
A 50 percent drop in the number of deaths from diabetes

Now you know what to eat to keep your body in top running condition. And you can look forward to learning to taste all manner of exquisite and subtly scrumptious foods. In terms of food, you have the ability to become a child again.

22

The Age-Old Secret Of Losing Weight

THERE is one overriding, outstanding, and painfully obvious "secret" to losing weight. Eat less.

That's almost all there is to it. The full secret is only slightly longer: eat less of the bad food and more of the good. If you kept on eating the same amount of food as you did before getting this book, but you switched from foods with fats, sugar, and sodium to foods with fiber, vitamins, and other nutrients (in other words, food from the four basic food groups), you would almost assuredly maintain your present weight and would probably even lose weight. This would happen without giving up the amount of food you are used to consuming. You'd definitely look and feel better even if you never lost a pound.

One funny thing about this method of weight loss—besides the fact that it's a secret known to every man, woman, and child in the modern world—is that the longer you remain on a healthy diet, the less food you'll need to satisfy your body's needs. One of the problems with junk food is that the lack of nutrients forces your body to demand more intake of food. Yes, eating bad foods can actually make you hungry sooner.

Even if you don't lose weight when you first switch over to healthy foods, as long as you continue the healthy eating habits you'll eventually lose weight and should reach your ideal weight. At which point you can slightly increase your protein and easily maintain your best weight.

So what's the problem?

Why do you suppose people don't make use of the age-old secret of losing weight? Why didn't you? Is it so hard to turn away from the bittersweet slow death of chocolate and turn toward the truly sweet soft juiciness of a fresh peach? Is it so difficult to refrain from indulging in the overkill of overly rich cookies and cakes and instead reach for the natural richness of whole wheat bread?

Well, yes. For some people it is very hard. And if you're one of them (or if you have a certain food that you cannot resist), you might be able to use some of the unusual methods of inducing weight loss or sustaining weight maintenance in this chapter. Before moving to these more intriguing techniques, let me point out that we're not talking about causing starvation (although some of you probably will swear that's what it feels like at first). We're really only outlining a way to help you choose the healthier foods.

Of course it sounds a bit boring: "eat your peas and carrots," "an apple a day," "protein plus dairy plus grain," and so on, but damn it, you *know* that it will work. The only reason you're still reading is that you're hoping for a miracle method of getting yourself to eat properly without having your taste patterns altered.

For, as you saw in the previous chapter, taste is what the fuss is about. People refuse to cut back on the saltiness of chips and dips. You see men and women at parties, standing near the rapidly diminishing mound of artificially flavored deep-fried potato skins, eager to gobble more and more of them with ever-increasing mounds of high-calorie toppings.

And people refuse to cut back on the sickly thick taste of alcohol. You see them pouring the stuff down their throats, adding fullness to their bellies without adding solid food to their systems.

And people refuse to cut back on the dreamy but deadly taste of creamy, sugary cakes. They sneak seconds at birthday parties or they grab another helping before the rush of blood sugar has even hit them in the first place.

Images of doom

I've deliberately used terms such as overkill, death, and deadly because the above-mentioned foods, while deliciously wicked fun in moderation, are contributing to your ultimate demise. You will die sooner than necessary if you're overweight. And while you're alive, you'll suffer from listlessness, a worrisome bloated feeling, fatigue, headaches, and self-recrimination.

Here's the bottom line on the bad foods: if you were on a desert island with a supply of candy and chocolate bars, you'd die. But substitute fresh fruit, water, and a small amount of protein and you'd live.

End of lecture. If you are up against a problem food, you might have to do something to fool your body, fool your mind, or fool your taste buds. I think I have that something.

The anti-eating shockers

Earlier in The Ego Diet, you saw how keeping certain images in your mind could help you refrain from overeating. You can think of yourself the way you intend to be at the end of your weight-loss period. You can use any reflective surface (including plates and silverware) to remind yourself to be careful of what you eat. You can keep a mental list of the foods you've already consumed during the day. You can hold a mental picture of someone you admire who you feel is at your ideal weight. And so on.

These mental methods will work, as you've seen if you've tried them. But sometimes you need something stronger. I am about to lead you through a personal anti-eating program, but you must promise to be extremely cautious about using it. You may not want to read all of it at once, but refer back to this section of the book from time to time over the next few months or years whenever you feel you need another anti-eating shocker (for that's what these items will be: shockers— deliberately designed to shock you into refraining from eating bad foods).

What will occur is an aversion conditioning process that is a self-administered behavior modification plan. This is something that you may or may not wish to do alone, but either way I recommend a discussion with a psychologist or psychiatrist before you undertake the program. Please proceed with caution.

Warning

Only if you cannot make yourself stop eating certain unhealthy foods should you attempt to use the examples in this section. If you have a handle on your eating habits, and the other Ego Diet methods are helping you, just skip to the Summary.

Some of the images that follow are repulsive and revolting. They are meant to be so. As a last resort method of preventing overeating, only a shocking image will be powerful enough to work.

Do not attempt to use more than one of these images at a time. The ugly and disturbing ideas that will be suggested to you are not meant to work in combination with one another. It will be better if you simply skip the entire section rather than read too much of it and get yourself into a bad state. By connecting disgusting images with certain foods, you can stop yourself from eating, but there is a very real danger in this method. You may become so turned off by these images that you get to the point where you are sickened by the act of eating. Therefore, you should only find the single image that works for you and associate it only with the food or foods that give you the most difficulty.

Care has been taken to place the less upsetting examples first so that the later ones have a greater intensity of effect. That way, you can read up to the point at which you no longer wish to associate perverse mental images with food. If the first couple of examples seem upsetting enough, by all means stop reading this section and skip ahead to the Summary.

An easy one

We'll begin with something simple and not too terribly upsetting, just to get the hang of it.

Let's say you're sitting and letting your mind wander for a moment. You could be at your desk while there's a slight lull in the day's activities. Or you could be at home on the couch watching television. Or any of a dozen places where you take time to think and plan.

All of a sudden, you think of food. Not just any food, but that special, extra-rich and creamy delicacy that always drives you crazy. This is the food that you cannot stop eating, so it is spoiling all of your best efforts with The Ego Diet. You begin salivating just imagining this particular food item. Your normal impulse at this point is to get up, go get some, and munch it.

Okay, go ahead. But while you're getting it and while you're eating it, think about the following things. Consider how this food is making you slow-moving. Like a sloth. Like a slug. Or like a snail. Imagine yourself as a wet snail each time you bite into the food.

Think about being inflated from the inside. The food is doing it. Each bite increases the pressure from within. You begin expanding, turning into a balloon. But a heavy, misshapen, lumpy balloon. Think about how all your clothes will have to be let out. Again. And now any new clothes you get will have to be made out of boat sails, because that's the only material large enough. Imagine the folds of your sleeves billowing out and flapping noisily in the breeze.

Think about how this food is making you loathsome and undesirable. Say the name of your problem food followed by the words "makes me ugly." Imagine how taking another bite of it would alter you physically. You'd see your skin shrivel up like the surface of a rotten piece of cactus.

Keep up these thoughts as long as you're thinking about (or eating) this food item. If the name, image, or idea of this food enters your mind, run through the above list of suggestions again. If one of them seems especially upsetting, repeat it.

Remember, only do this when you're thinking of the problem food. You don't have to think about these things at any other time. Just relax.

Snake in the grass

Or perhaps I should say snake in the hand. But before getting to that, consider whether the thought of snakes disturbs you. Of course, the thought of one isn't in and of itself frightening, although you may react in a frightened manner when confronted by a real one. Yet many people can send a shiver down their spine just remembering what the last snake they saw was doing when it scared them.

There are two theories of emotion that deal with the kind of reaction people sometimes have to snakes. The first, the James-Lange theory, states that seeing something like a snake provokes an internal reaction —your heart pounds faster, your stomach tenses, and so on—and this, in turn, causes an emotional response, namely fear. The Cannon-Bard theory, however, holds that we experience the emotional response at the same time we experience the physical reactions. The Cannon-Bard theory seems more correct until there is an accident, when we tend to act physically even before any emotions begin reaching the surface. But whichever theory is closer to the truth, the fact remains that some images produce more violent reactions than others, and that the reactions are both emotional and physical in the long run. It is this fact that causes the next suggestion to work. However, if snakes do not frighten you, then you should do one of two things. Either skip to the next example (if you're ready for it) or try to use the following images in a way that suits an animal that frightens you. Some people are afraid of dogs. Some of horses. Some of insects. Use whatever scares you.

Imagine holding a snake in your hands while eating your problem food. (Let's say the food you have trouble with is chocolate fudge— we'll use this as an example from now on.)

Think about holding a long, green, rapidly twitching snake. Imagine it coiled around your plate of fudge. Think about biting into the fudge and finding a snake inside. Or half a snake.

(Obviously, if your fear is dogs, that last example isn't likely to work. However, you can think of a conceptual art exhibit I once saw in which observers walked between two cages so close together you had to move sideways. In each cage—in front of you and behind you—was an attack-trained Doberman guard dog. Both dogs charged the side of the cage near you, snarling and growling, and followed you through the passageway. Once you were inside, there was nowhere to go but through the exhibit. Think about being inside that environment every time you think about fudge.)

The sleeping serpent

Yes, we're back on the subject of snakes. This time, you're going to become a snake. Really. Close your eyes while thinking of a big plate of fudge and see yourself covered with rippling, interlocked scales. Because of that fudge, your body has become a long, squirming tube, wriggling in the dirt.

This analogy isn't too farfetched. Gobbling up food is an animalistic reaction. You've probably noticed how dogs and cats will sometimes chow down on their favorite food like it will be their last meal for the week. They only stop to burp.

Now imagine yourself as one of those gargantuan snakes you've seen in the zoo or in jungle movies. You slither through the underbrush quietly and carefully until you come upon a family of wild pigs. You slide forward suddenly, scattering most of them. You quickly wrap your huge body around one of the squealing piglets. The squeals get harsh and high, then abruptly end as you crush the air out of its lungs. It struggles as you stretch open your mouth and force it down your very long throat.

When you put fudge into your body, consider the image of yourself as a snake sunning itself with a bloated, distended belly that is full of half-digested baby pig.

Plates full of fire

What if touching fudge scorched your fingers? Think about it being able to cause fires inside you or on your skin. Just getting near the chocolate makes you think of the sheets of heat you feel at a forest fire. Your temperature soars. You hear the crackling of timber and brush burning. The sound builds to a roar as the wall of fire gets closer.

As you reach for the fudge, it's like striking a match while covered with gasoline. You burst into flame.

Elephants have the most

I once attended the circus at the Forum in Inglewood, California. This is the basketball arena used by the Los Angeles Lakers, so it is a large place. During the parade of elephants, about two dozen of them walked or ran around the track between the spectators and the three inner performance rings. While moving around the track, some of the pachyderms do what you have no doubt seen horses do during a parade: they lifted their tails and let go of the largest amount of excrement you've ever imagined could be held in one beast. Patrons who happened to be sitting in the front rows, on the same level with the elephants, made a hasty retreat, provoking laughter from many of the fans seated above them. One spectator called out "Chicken!" which made a few return to their seats. The rest remained in the aisles, milling around awkwardly. But they were the smart ones.

As the next part of the elephants' routine, they stopped moving around the track and instead each spun slowly around in the space where it stood. While this made for an awesome sight for those of us high enough up to appreciate it, there was one minor drawback for the front rows: as the big animals swung their ponderous bodies around, their posteriors came even closer to the front rows. From where I was seated, it looked as if those people in the first five rows had a proctologist's-eye view of the north end of several southbound elephants.

Now the elephants are all facing the center of the arena while shifting their weight from one front leg to the other. This has the effect of swinging their hindquarters back and forth, bringing peals of laughter from the crowd. But again, the rumps of the beasts were coming close to those in the front rows. Very close. Too close.

The thought struck many of us in the audience at the same time: what if one of the elephants lets go now? A curious, expectant hush gradually fell over us, contrasting mightily with the tinny amplified music of the circus band.

The tension became palpable as we waited and watched. Would it happen? Could it happen? Do you suppose, if just one of the elephants —there! That one! And that one, too! The people down there had better watch it or they're going to get covered with. . . . Yup, they got covered with it.

Excrement almost always provokes nervous laughter. This is something we learn from parents and peers when growing up—that it is an embarrassing subject, and one fit for humor. Yet at the same time we also learn revulsion for excrement. While this is hardly the most enlightened approach to the subject, it is true in this society, neverthe- less. And it affords us the opportunity to picture fudge on a platter surrounded by human excrement and a choice selection of animal excrement, steaming hot.

Have you ever heard the phrase, "Eat s—— and die"? Just think about doing that. Consider it being in your hands and nibbling it along with the fudge.

For some reason, this particular anti-eating shocker works quite well with chocolate, éclairs, and sausages. (See, I told you this subject produced nervous laughter.)

Primal fears

Certain phobias, or fears, seem more common than others. The fears that many people share, and which extend back to early childhood, are sometimes called primal fears. These can include the fear of fire, water, falling, closed-in spaces, heights, and wide-open spaces (frequently coupled with height). Any of these, like the suggestions regarding fire, may be used to help you battle the cravings for certain foods.

Although fire is something that we can all appreciate as a phobia, some of the others may not have any shock value to many of us. Only a person with a fear of being in a closed-in space can make good use of the suggestion to associate fudge with being in an elevator that starts to get smaller while the doors are jammed shut, or with the idea of being inside a coffin and buried in the earth (although death may represent an excellent fear to begin associating with your particular problem food).

Only you know if one of these phobias is shocking enough to work well for you.

Creepy crawlies

When an animal dies in the wilderness and the insects, wolves, buzzards, or rats don't get to the body in time to devour it before the flesh turns foul, a curious sort of beast is born. The flies that swarm over the rotting meat produce larvae: soft-bodied, footless, wormlike creatures. They will become flies in time, but in this state, hundreds or even thousands of them wriggle and squirm their way in and out of the decaying body of the dead animal. Picture this in your mind when the thought of fudge occurs to you.

The sickening little garbage disposal units are called maggots. A mass of maggots on a carcass can look like an undulating white pile of lumpy spit. Think of them crawling on your fudge.

If this example doesn't turn you away from your problem food, there's only one more image that could possibly have an effect.

Meat on the hoof

You are moving slowly through a long wooden chute. There is no room to turn to the left or right. The line of cows jammed tightly up against one another moves inexorably forward. Stragglers are kept jumping forward by herders who reach through the wooden boards with cattle prods—long-handled electrical devices that send a jolt of energy through the skin of any animal they touch.

There is a smell of death in the air, and the animals are lowing restlessly. As the line approaches the slaughterhouse, a sound that had been merely a dull thud now becomes clear and distinct. First, there is a quick hiss of air as a big metal piston is sent zooming down its cylinder housing. At the end of the cylinder, the piston head protrudes with violent force where it meets up with . . .

The skull of the adult cow is larger than that of a human, and constructed along different lines. Yet it is still just an interlocking set of bones with a movable jaw. When the killing piston blow slams into the top of the animal's skull, there is a cracking, smashing crunch. Blood flies through the air in little arcs as the body of the beast collapses to the floor.

The gallons of blood inside the cow must be drained away, so the animal is slit open while the body is still warm. The red juice flows through sluice gates, then the dead animal is skinned and dismembered and quickly turned into large hunks of meat we later know as rib roast, steak, roast beef, and so on.

The death knell of the hammer hitting heads continues hour after hour in the slaughterhouse—one of many in Los Angeles, Chicago, Kansas City, and other large metropolitan centers. Day in and day out, the killing goes on, supervised by men in blood-soaked rain boots and slickers. We must have this killing in order to stock the supermarket shelves with beef. And the pork products require the same sort of killing of hogs.

If you bring this image of death and bloodletting to your mind's eye when you have the urge to eat something bad for you, I hope the feeling of sadness is enough to make you stop. And if it helps you avoid the fatty meats as well, so much the better.

Summary

I didn't intend the anti-eating shockers to be such a revolting experience that you'd have difficulty dealing with all food. Which is why I stressed the fact that you should not read all of the examples at once.

That could result in an image overload. If you made this mistake, my sympathies. Please look around you for some sweetness and light: a child playing, a flower blooming, a friend or lover smiling at you. These things should be what we live for. The ugly images are nothing more than tools to make The Ego Diet work perfectly for you.

I would like to leave you with four thoughts from the many points made in this book. First, The Ego Diet is not something you should use to speed up your weight loss. It is a slow weight-loss plan, and one of the best weight-maintenance plans ever devised.

Second, because it enables you to reach inside yourself and draw on the power of your own ego, this plan is self-actualizing and self-perpetuating. You can find sources of resolve and dynamism you never knew you possessed. You have the ability to take full control of your own life, and you can keep changing your part of the world every single day. You know you'll be better for it, and because you are the world will be better too.

Third, The Ego Diet is as concerned with good nutrition and good health as it is with weight loss. Remember, you may be at your ideal weight despite being a few pounds heavier than some weight chart recommends—and it is far healthier simply to remain a few pounds "overweight" rather than to lose the pounds, gain them back, lose them, gain, and so forth.

Fourth, you can use the methods in The Ego Diet to help you win the many small battles in your own private war against foods high in fat, sugar, and sodium. You only have to fight off the temptation right at the moment it strikes. You don't have to worry about later on, or tomorrow, or the next month—just find an Ego Diet method that works *right now*. Because you can't lose weight or maintain weight in the future, you can only do it at the present moment. Win each tiny battle and the war will take care of itself.

The happy ending

You control the outcome of more than this book. You control the outcome of your life. You've been both hero and villain during the course of reading *The Ego Diet*. Now, it's time to stride out into your life and be the hero for good.

You can do it. You know it. You can feel it.

Be your own hero.

Glossary

addiction.   A physical and/or psychological dependence on drugs, alcohol, or
  food. It almost always involves excessive and persistent use of the substances. You are addicted to a substance if you experience withdrawal
  symptoms (intense craving, nervous shakes, or obsessive consumption of
  substitute items) when you no longer have the substance.
adrenaline.   A hormone that is secreted when your body is confronted by
  frightening or stressful situations. It is adrenaline that gives you a quick-
  ened pulse when you're about to speak before a group of people. The
  actual name of this hormone is epinephrine; Adrenalin is the trade name
  for a synthetic substance, but so common is its use, the two terms are
  becoming synonomous.
anorexia nervosa (anorexia).   Abnormal, prolonged loss of appetite or an
  aversion to food. This is a psychoneurotic disorder. Unlike a psychosis,
  which is a break with reality, a psychoneurosis represents an attempt by
  the individual to resolve some inner conflict. People who become
  anorexic are literally starving themselves to death (although often the
  victim dies of illnesses brought on by a weakened condition, as in the
  case of singer Karen Carpenter).
anti-eating shockers.   Disturbing images that, when brought to mind, will
  discourage the eating of certain foods.
approach-avoidance conflict.   The problem faced by people whose desires
  conflict with reality. This occurs, for example, when you want to eat a
  piece of pie but you don't want to add any calories to your diet.
association areas.   Those higher parts of your brain with extremely complex
  connections between neurons, and presumed to deal with our more complicated mental functions: learning, memory, and thinking.
aversive conditioning.   As in the use of the anti-eating shockers in Chapter 22,
  you associate an unpleasant sensation (such as phobias: fear of snakes,
  water, fire, etc.) with a certain kind of food so as to diminish your desire
  for that food.

behavior modification.   A means of altering someone's actions by rewarding
  the desired behavior and/or punishing the undesired behavior.
binge-purge cycle.   Overeating followed by prolonged aversion to food or by
  vomiting to rid the body of food.
blood-sugar level.   The amount of sugar in your blood. When it gets too low,
  your body signals you to feel hunger.
bulimia.   Being hungry all the time; a constant craving for food. From the
  French *bous* (cow head) and *limos* (hunger).

central nervous system.   The brain and the spinal cord functioning together.

classical conditioning.   This is the one Pavlov discovered after experimenting with his dogs. An unnatural stimulus is associated with a natural one (in the case of Pavlov's dogs, a bell was rung just as food was given to them; eventually, the dogs would salivate at the sound of the bell, without food being present).

conditioned response.   The salivating of Pavlov's dogs was a conditioned response. Because the stimulus (the bell) had been so carefully and closely associated with an action (being fed), a response was "built in" for the dogs.

diet.   The totality of what you eat, when you eat it, how fast you eat it, and how much of it you eat. Everyone is on a diet. The goal of The Ego Diet is for you to control your diet.

ectomorph.   A person with a thin body.

ego.   The Freudian term for the controlling mechanism in your personality that balances the desires of the id and the reservations of the superego while checking on the reactions of people and events outside the self.

endomorph.   A person with a fat body.

glands.   Various organs inside your body which start chemical changes and reactions so that specific tasks may be carried out. Digestion of food, for example, triggers many glandular actions.

habituation.   Becoming accustomed to the effects of continued consumption of a drug, alcohol, or food; a "habit."

hedonism.   One of the theories of motivation. This one, apparent in the actions of most people around us, holds that we seek pleasurable experiences and avoid unpleasant ones.

hierarchy of needs.   Maslow's theory that basic needs (shelter, food, safety, etc.) must be met before higher needs (acceptance in a group, feelings of self-worth, etc.) can be dealt with.

hypothalamus.   A portion of the brain which regulates hunger, thirst, and some emotions.

id.   The Freudian term for the part of your personality concerned with satisfying basic desires (or even base desires).

mesomorph. A person with an athletic body.

neuron. The basic nerve cell. Information is transmitted within your body by chemical/electrical messages between neurons.

oral stage. A stage in a person's development when the mouth is of primary importance.

peers. Members of your own social, business, and/or age group.

repression. The wiping out of conscious thought on a certain topic. Or, the denying of certain thoughts or impulses.

self-actualization. The developmental level that should be everyone's goal: this capacity for the fullest expression of life is attained when a person is in control of his or her needs.

spinal cord. This is a kind of automatic brain that sends messages to all parts of your body.

superego. Like your conscience; in Freudian terms, it is the warning center.

tolerance. The body's ability to adapt to the dosage of a drug or alcohol, which often leads to a person increasing the dosage.